Herbal Exchanges

in celebration of the
National Institute of Medical Herbalists
1864–2014

FRANCES WATKINS

at Biophilia II 9/3/19

THE NATIONAL INSTITUTE
OF MEDICAL
HERBALISTS
1864 - 2014

First published in Great Britain by Strathmore Publishing,
41 Kingsway Place, Sans Walk, London EC1R 0LU, 2014
on behalf of the National Institute of Medical Herbalists, Clover House, James Court,
South Street, Exeter, Devon, EX1 1EE

978-1-909277-08-3

Disclaimer

No responsibility is assumed by the NIMH or the publisher for any injury and/or damage to persons or property as a matter of products liability, negligence or otherwise, or from any use or operation of any methods, products, instructions or ideas contained in the material herein. Because of rapid advances in the medical sciences, in particular, independent verification of diagnoses and drug dosages should be made.

Views and opinions expressed in this book do not necessarily reflect those of the National Institute of Medical Herbalists and the editorial team.

Design and origination by Strathmore Publishing Ltd. London
Typeset in RotisSerif and RotisSansSerif
Printed in England by Berforts Information Press, The Old School House,
Castle Rising, King's Lynn, Norfolk, PE31 6AG

Herbal Exchanges

in celebration of the
National Institute of Medical Herbalists
1864–2014

edited by Hananja Brice-Ytsma
and Frances Watkins

STRATHMORE PUBLISHING
LONDON
2014

Contents

Foreword

Dr Michael Dixon

A very happy birthday to the National Institute of Medical Herbalists. The survival of any Institution for 150 years is an achievement in its own right but medical herbalists, as these pages will reveal, are a very special breed indeed!

I have also regarded herbal medicine as medicine in colour. Medicine that connects us to the earth through its healing plants and medicine, whose wisdom often goes far back in time. As an NHS GP, I have been interested in herbal medicine for a number of years and not only because it is utterly fascinating but because it also works.

An increasing number of herbal medicines are now proven to work beyond reasonable doubt. The introduction of the Traditional Herb Directive in April 2011 also means that herbal medicines are safe and often safer than conventional medicines, which have a shorter history. In my own surgery, we did a trial a few years ago, when all the partners offered patients with five specific problems such as poor sleep, the choice of conventional or herbal remedy. Patients tended to prefer the herbal alternative, most were helped by it and a significant number said they would buy a herbal remedy in future before seeing the GP. Herbal medicine has an enormous potential role in health service sustainability.

Of course, herbal medicine goes far beyond doctors suggesting patients buying herbal medicines over the counter. Medical herbalists are the alchemists of mother nature's gift. This not only involves detailed knowledge of the herbs themselves but also an ability to individualise treatment centred on each patient in a way that conventional medicine has sometimes forgotten. Increasingly, conventional medicine is moving from giving patients a substantial dose of one drug to giving small amounts of many. In hypertension or cancer, for instance, this leads to maximum effect but with minimum side effects. These are things that medical herbalists have known for many years and the skill is in getting the right mix of the right herbs for the right patient.

One can only hope on this 150th anniversary that the professional divide between conventional clinicians and medical herbalists will come to an end. It is a divide that has too often used spurious arguments to conceal vested interest. The hoped for statutory regulation of medical herbalists alongside conventional medicine taking on a broader perspective should help this. So too should the drive towards helping patients to help themselves, personalise medicine and the need to create a sustainable health service that conserves expensive technology and hospitals for only when they are absolutely necessary. Medical herbalists will be playing a major role in this new world less because other clinicians or politicians allow them to do so and more because patients will demand it. After all they have been integrating their care between different clinicians for many years and it is on their behalf that we clinicians must now join forces to provide an integrated service for our patients that forgets the divides and the disputes of the past.

Finally, I want to thank all those medical herbalists, who have seen my patients over the past thirty years. Almost universally they have been helped, almost universally they have reported their experience as positive and holistic and almost universally they have improved their general resilience. Would that every clinician could say the same!

Introduction

Laura Stannard
President, National Institute of Medical Herbalists

Significant birthdays and anniversaries are often times when we reflect on events that have shaped our lives, the paths we have followed, the milestones we have encountered along the way, our achievements and things we are proud of, as well as things we might wish had been even slightly different. They are also times for looking forward with hope for the future and what it may bring.

As we, the current members of the National Institute of Medical Herbalists, mark the 150th anniversary of the founding of our organisation, we invite all our friends and colleagues from sister organisations around the world to share this occasion for we are all involved in herbal medicine and connected by our passion for the healing power of herbs and together we can celebrate a significant event in the world of herbal medicine.

Herbal medicine is common to all civilisations and all peoples throughout the world. Why then, has it been such a struggle for the oldest and commonest form of medicine to find a place in what might be called 'approved' healthcare?

In the1850s a group of herbalists met to bring together the various herbalists working at that time with the aim of forming a society for the furtherance of the studies into herbal medicines; thus in 1864 the National Association of Medical Herbalists (NAMH) was formed, 'dedicated to encourage the study and knowledge of the vegetable kingdom and its application to public health'.

Following the Second World War, in 1945, the name was changed, to the National Institute of Medical Herbalists (NIMH) forming one large national unified body for all unregistered practice in medicine.

Since its inception the history of, first, the NAMH as it was, later the NIMH, has been peppered with struggles to overcome attempts at passing legislation which would restrict the activity of the herbalist and the people's choice of medical treatment.

For 150 years the NIMH has led the struggle to achieve recognition of the part herbal medicine plays in healthcare. Throughout those 150 years herbalists have encountered various Acts of Parliament and pieces of legislation, which now includes legislation from the European Union (EU) that have threatened the practice of herbal medicine. Herbalists have had to fight for their very existence and our patients have had to fight alongside us just to exercise their choice of treatment.

The 1941 Medicines Bill was hurriedly passed despite the world being at war; it effectively outlawed the practice of herbal medicine. However herbs were hugely significant – even as late as the 1930s up to 90 per cent of drugs used in Britain were derived from plants, most of which were imported from continental Europe. The war meant there was a shortage of essential drugs. The Vegetable Drugs Committee was formed and people were called upon to gather herbal medicines from the wild and grow them in gardens. However the herbs collected were not intended to be used as whole plants; the constituents were removed to manufacture drugs. Meanwhile herbalists such as Albert Orbell continued to work despite the war and legislation.

Following the thalidomide tragedy of the 1960s, the UK government sought to introduce legislation requiring testing and licensing of all medicines and herbal medicines, as well as an embargo on dispensing tinctures, fluid extracts and ointments. The NIMH swung into action. Fred Fletcher Hyde the NIMH president at the time, led the campaign tirelessly. Members, patients, users of herbal medicine and supporters deluged MPs and the Department of Health with letters. Fred spent so much time in the House of Lords negotiating amendments to the legislation that he was frequently greeted by staff there as "M'lud". A major victory was won in the end and for the first time there was a legal basis for herbal practice with a clause inserted into the 1968 Medicine's Act (Section 12i). It is not an exaggeration to say that herbalists in the UK owe our current ability to practise to the tireless work of Fred Fletcher Hyde.

From the beginning, the NAMH and then the NIMH has sought to provide a unified voice for the herbal profession. The NAMH began by bringing together herbalists, and in the years that followed the founding of the NAMH botanical medicine societies across Britain joined. The change of name in 1945 came as a result of the need to speak with one voice. In 1994, when yet another struggle to maintain the right to practise herbal medicine and provide the UK population with choice ensued, the NIMH spearheaded another campaign. Once a solution was found to the immediate problem, the NIMH council brought together the other herbal associations and traditions including Ayurveda and Traditional Chinese Medicine to create an umbrella body, the European Herbal Practitioners Association (EHPA), which would speak for herbal medicine in all the modalities now practised in the UK. The NIMH had begun forming the EHPA a year earlier but events in 1994 showed how important it was to draw the other herbalists together with a common aim. From the beginning, the EHPA was headed up by Michael McIntyre, a former NIMH president, who for over 20 years has been the driving force behind the organisation which seeks to maintain access for the public to safe and effective herbal treatment at the hands of recognised and qualified professionals from every herbal tradition now found in the UK.

The vision of herbal medicine taking its rightful place in healthcare is carried forward to today. In the UK we had almost crossed the finish line when in February 2011 the Heath Secretary, Andrew Lansley announced there would be Statutory Regulation of herbalists – almost but not quite. Three years after that announcement, when we should be celebrating our 150th anniversary with a legal basis for the practice of herbal medicine, we see further attempts to stop regulation happening. At the time of writing, the government has convened another Working Group to look at whether or not herbalists should be regulated by statute. While the UK government deliberates on whether or not to recognise herbal medicine practice, the World Health Organisation seeks to integrate traditional herbal medicine into the healthcare systems of all member countries (See WHO Traditional Medicine Strategy 2014–2023). I hope that the recommendation of the Working Group will be a resounding 'Yes' and herbalists will become an integral part of the UK's healthcare system.

In order to take that place in healthcare, herbal medicine practitioners must be educated and trained to the highest possible standards. Throughout the NAMH and NIMH history, provision for education and training of herbalists has been hugely important and is one of the Objects in the Articles of Association. Independent schools have been established although none survive, including the College of Herbal Medicine in Southport created by William Henry Webb, the College of

Botanic Medicine in London, the School of Herbal Medicine in Tunbridge Wells (which became the College of Phytotherapy and moved to Bodle Street Green) and the Scottish School of Herbal Medicine pioneered by Keith and Maureen Robertson.

In September 1994, education in herbal medicine took on a new dimension. Middlesex University in collaboration with NIMH, opened its doors to the first cohort of herbal students in the world to take a BSc (Hons) degree in Herbal Medicine and paved the way for several other universities to follow suit. The NIMH was aware that these undergraduate courses needed to be open to public scrutiny, as well as meeting appropriate educational requirements. In 1996 the NIMH Accreditation Board was officially launched and comprised members of the herbal profession and lay members drawn from higher education and health related fields.

The NIMH is no stranger to innovation. Whether it is the establishment of an independent Accreditation Board to oversee standards in education, the creation of an internationally recognised academic journal, introducing mandatory Continuing Professional Development for all members, developing a mentor scheme for newly qualified practitioners, working with university departments, embracing technology and social media, devising rigorous procedures to allow colleagues who have trained differently to take their place in our ranks, the NIMH has led the way.

One of the aims of the NIMH is the creation and maintenance of a library. The purchase of an office in Exeter in 2011 has provided a permanent space where a library could be housed.

Throughout herbal history and the history of the NIMH books have been written. Whether it is the ancient work of Dioscorides or the recent work of Kerry Bone and Simon Mills, books crystallise the knowledge of herbal practice at any given moment. In any field books make and establish a profession, giving it identity and describing the professional knowledge that sets that profession apart. In the last 150 years, the works of John Skelton, Albert Priest and Lillian Priest and Thomas Bartram have described and distilled herbal practice, while recent works such as Mills and Bone have explored research into herbal medicine and herbal medicines. Peter Conway has investigated what occurs in the act of consultation, an under-researched and often overlooked area even in mainstream circles. Graeme Tobyn, Alison Denham and Midge Whitelegg have examined the tradition of herbal medicine through the medicines themselves. Elsewhere in the world the likes of Ruth Trickey, David Winston, Mathew Wood and Stephen Harrod Buhner have advanced the knowledge of herbal practice sharing clinical experience.

The NIMH library is being added to year by year, not only with classical texts but with new publications from amongst our contemporaries. Legacies have helped stock the library shelves. Donations are welcome.

Surviving 150 years is no mean feat. Maintaining an organisation for 150 years requires the same vision that founded it, coupled with dedication and determination. Could it be that the NIMH has reached 150 years because of the storms it has had to weather?

The Eden Project in Cornwall, in the southwest of England, is an attempt to build a perfect environment in which plants and trees would flourish. Huge domes, called biomes, provide a closely monitored atmosphere with a perfect temperature range and humidity and there is no pollution. What more could a tree want?

The project encountered a problem. The scientists noticed the leaves on the big trees were beginning to wilt and the branches were starting to droop. A tree expert was called in, and told them the problem is that there is no wind in the environment of the biomes. It is the wind that pushes and moves the tree fibres forcing the nutrients and moisture to be drawn up from the ground causing nutrients to reach where they are needed and the trunk to become strong. Trees need the stress of the wind or they will not thrive. No tree can grow strong unless there is an occasional storm; even a strong breeze might be sufficient.

Let us hope that the future brings gentler breezes for the NIMH, just strong enough to keep us as robust as we have been up to now and need to be to continue for the next 150 years while we endeavour to fulfil the aims of our founders and the objects of the NIMH namely to 'promote and encourage the study and practice, with a view to the relief of human suffering, of the art and science of Medical Herbalism'.

In the March 1964 issue of *The Herbal Practitioner* marking the NIMH centenary the author (unknown) of the outline history of the NIMH wrote:

> *'A society struggling for its rights, and having to continually fight for its very existence, with no state grants for education of its students or for research into its medicaments is not in a very satisfactory position, and it is a credit to the long past members of the Association councils that the herbal profession was indeed maintained at such remarkably high standards.'*

Fifty years on we can say the same things. We can look on that as an indictment of those in our society who for whatever reason fail or refuse to acknowledge the role herbal medicine plays, or we can look at it as another fifty years of endeavour, keeping alive our medical tradition, and taking it forward, developing it, and working to ensure that all future generations will have the choice to be treated by herbalists and to become herbalists. After 150 years we are as passionate and dedicated as we have always been. We have seen our profession develop, overcome many obstacles, and flourish.

The legacy of our forebears John Skelton, William Fox, William Henry Webb, as well as the likes of Fred Fletcher Hyde, Albert and Lillian Priest, Hein Zeylstra and Michael Mcintyre who have continued to further herbal practice in more recent times is immeasurable. None of us would be practising today had it not been for them, and the others like them, past and present. Alongside each one of them stands every member of the NIMH who has as an individual devoted themselves to the practice of herbal medicine and the relief of human suffering – every single member for 150 years, whether their name is well recognised and known or not is a hero of herbal medicine. Quietly going about the business of caring for patients, the members of the NIMH have embodied herbal medicine for 150 years.

Acknowledgements

The idea for this book came from Hananja Brice-Ytsma, NIMH Director of Education. Hananja wanted to find a unique and memorable way to celebrate the 150th anniversary of the founding of the National Institute of Medical Herbalists. The result is this book: an expression of the diversity of interest, thought and practice of Western medical herbalism from leading practitioners in the UK and across the world. All of the contributors have been gracious with their time, and offered us this wonderful eclectic mix of enlightening material. The personal insights are intended to appeal to readers of all levels of herbal experience and all those with an interest in herbal medicine.

Such a project would not be complete without expressing gratitude to all those who have helped bring it to fruition.

Our sincere thanks to all contributors without whom the pages of this book would have remained blank. In reaching out to our colleagues across the world, we hope to have created a new era for herbal medicine, one where our common passion can bring us together as individuals, colleagues and professional associations, proud of our uniqueness and our heritage, and united by our shared experience of enabling healing through the use of medicinal plants. Herbal medicine has a bright future; let us create it together as NIMH has created this book.

We are hugely appreciative to Marion MacKonochie and Caroline Sheldrick for copy editing, Frances Hambly and Cheryl Reynolds for proof reading and for the giving of their time; Elspeth McPherson from Strathmore Publishing for coordinating the print and book production; Penny Price for the pen drawing of dandelion on the front cover and to Kay Piercy for the beautiful plant images that introduce each section.

Lastly and perhaps most importantly, an enormous thank you to the editors of the book: Frances Watkins who assisted from the very earliest days, embracing the idea with drive and enthusiasm and helped make sure the project came to fruition; and to Hananja herself, whose vision is now made manifest in what you hold in your hands.

Thank you one and all.

NIMH Council 2014

Herbal Heritage

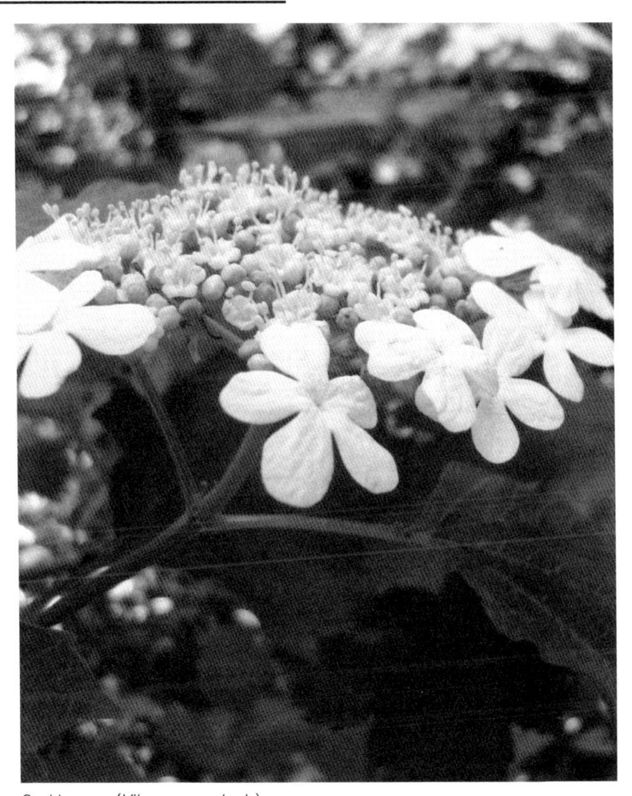

Guelder-rose (*Viburnum opulus* L.)

A brief history of the National Institute of Medical Herbalists

Desiree Shelley

The focus of this article is to highlight a number of milestones in the history of the formation of the National Institute of Medical Herbalists. In the first half of the 19th century herbalists continued to practise under the protection of the Herbalists Charter enacted by Henry VIII in 1542 (MacLennan and Pendry 2011). Albert Isaiah Coffin came to England in 1838 bringing the Thomsonian system of Botanic Practice of Medicine from America. Coffin travelled around the country teaching medical botany, setting up medico-botanical societies, many in the north of England, and appointing herbalists as agents to sell his herbal remedies and books to the public.

The Medical Act of 1858 created a statutory register of licensed practitioners and established The General Medical Council to oversee training and standards of medical practice. The purpose of this Act was to distinguish qualified from unqualified medical practitioners (MacLennan and Pendry 2011). In the same year a group of Medical-Botanic Practitioners met in Manchester with the aim of forming a united society, and so the British Medico Botanic Society was formed, later incorporating the British Medical Reform Association and was the foundation of the National Association of Medical Herbalists (NAMH) (NAMH 1908).

The Apothecaries Act of 1815, section 20, allowed prosecution against herbalists for example, a James Wallis practising in London was tried in 1884 for manslaughter by a Coroner's jury for poisoning with lobelia. At the trial, a party of NAMH members appeared as witnesses resulting in a verdict of not guilty. Council members were also instrumental in preventing lobelia from being included in the Poison Schedule: 'if the existence of the NAMH has secured no other benefit to its members this alone would repay all fees ever paid in reserving to herbalists so valuable a remedy as lobelia.' (NAMH 1908)

The core aims of NAMH were to study and research herbal medicine, to teach and expound herbal knowledge, to practise and promote awareness of its members and the Association. In 1887 NAMH published The *Botanic Practitioner and Journal of the National Association of Medical Herbalists of Great Britain* for members and students. NAMH was registered as a company limited by guarantee in 1895 under the presidency of Alfred Russell Fox. The NAMH Council formed sub-committees from 1901 for examination of prospective new members, parliamentary activity, publishing and education of new herbalists (NAMH 1901).

A number of NAMH members travelled to America to exchange herbal knowledge and experiences and as a result, new plants entered into the British herbal dispensaries for example echinacea (*Echinacea angustifolia* DC.) and cimicifuga (*Cimicifuga racemosa* (L.) Nutt.). Likewise, American herbalists were arriving in England and setting up practice. William H Webb started a School of Herbal Medicine at 11 Scarisbrick Street, in Southport with his American born wife Dr Sarah Webb, in 1902. NAMH invested in the school which included a sanatorium and was named 'The Botanic Sanatorium and Training School of the NAMH of GB Ltd.' It became the new Herbalists Medical College in 1911 and was officially opened by the herbalist Alderman Henry Potter (NAMH 1902, 1911).

NAMH Council drafted a Herbalist Bill in 1902 and spent the next

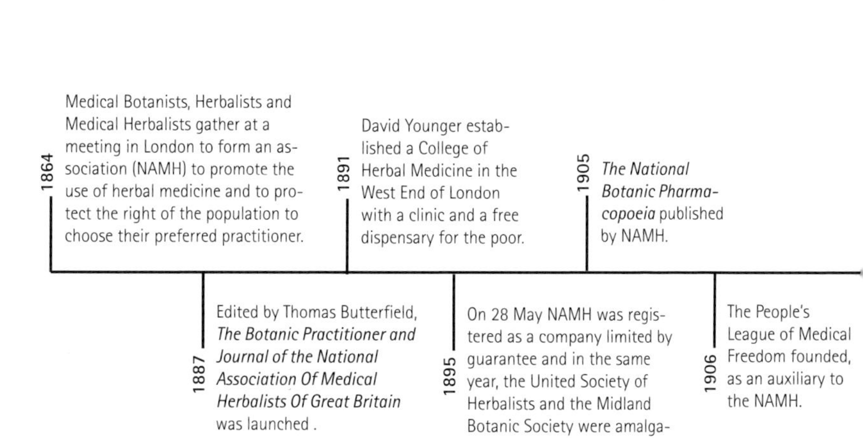
1864
Medical Botanists, Herbalists and Medical Herbalists gather at a meeting in London to form an association (NAMH) to promote the use of herbal medicine and to protect the right of the population to choose their preferred practitioner.
1887
Edited by Thomas Butterfield, *The Botanic Practitioner and Journal of the National Association Of Medical Herbalists Of Great Britain* was launched .
1891
David Younger established a College of Herbal Medicine in the West End of London with a clinic and a free dispensary for the poor.
1895
On 28 May NAMH was registered as a company limited by guarantee and in the same year, the United Society of Herbalists and the Midland Botanic Society were amalgamated into NAMH.
1905
The National Botanic Pharmacopoeia published by NAMH.
1906
The People's League of Medical Freedom founded, as an auxiliary to the NAMH.

twenty years promoting it with Members of Parliament, Herbalists and the general public. The Bill was eventually introduced into Parliament in 1923 with the support of 130 MPs. It was read for the first time without opposition, but due to it being a Private Members' Bill and not a Government measure it was subsequently dropped. (NAMH 1902, 1923).

The National Insurance Act of 1911 was one of the strongest blows to the continued existence of herbal medicine. The NAMH secretary reported 'the handing over to the absolute mercy of the allopaths of about 15 millions of people, without any appeal against their decision, is a most serious matter.' Prior to the inception of the new State Medical Service, Mr A Bevin, the then Minister of Health, received a deputation of herbalists whose object it was to press the claim for State recognition; once again this did not happen. When the National Health Service started in 1948, NIMH and the Hospital of Natural Healing in East London came together to found the School of Herbal Medicine, offering students the facilities for clinical training and instruction on a par with the outpatients department of orthodox hospitals (NIMH 1948).

The 100th NIMH conference was held at the Guildhall in London 30-31 March1964 and presided over by Mr Albert Orbell. The Vice-President Mr Arthur Jenner gave a lecture titled 'The Future of Herbal Medicine' and was so well received that it was published in *The Herbal Practitioner* to share with all members. One opening statement is poignant even today: 'The future worth and social status of medical herbalism will be directly proportional to the vision, energy and action shown by the present members'. He then went on to say:

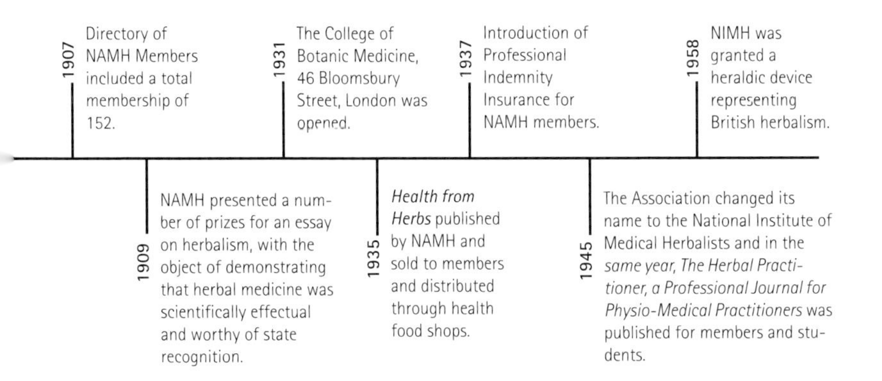

1907
Directory of NAMH Members included a total membership of 152.
1909
NAMH presented a number of prizes for an essay on herbalism, with the object of demonstrating that herbal medicine was scientifically effectual and worthy of state recognition.
1931
The College of Botanic Medicine, 46 Bloomsbury Street, London was opened.
1935
Health from Herbs published by NAMH and sold to members and distributed through health food shops.
1937
Introduction of Professional Indemnity Insurance for NAMH members.
1945
The Association changed its name to the National Institute of Medical Herbalists and in the same year, The Herbal Practitioner, a Professional Journal for Physio-Medical Practitioners was published for members and students.
1958
NIMH was granted a heraldic device representing British herbalism.

'The basis of any learned society is education. The education of our students, and the elevation of our academic standards must eventually secure the true recognition of our methods. There must be a good basic groundwork in Biology, Anatomy, Physiology and Pathology, yet without undue pedantry... We must teach a sound knowledge of physiomedical philosophy, materia medica and therapeutics. The physical technique but provides a physical rapport with the patient, whilst Psychotherapy based on the simple 'common-sense' approach lays the foundations for a psychosomatic orientation to health and disease. Efficiency in practical clinical diagnostic procedure is regarded as absolutely essential, as also the confidence and ability to apply good physiomedicalism, both of which will depend upon adequate practical training and clinical experience. In this respect, the Hospital for Natural Healing is already being used, and will be increasingly so used in the future' (Jenner, 1964)

NIMH has throughout its history published journals for the membership and in 1935 produced *Health from Herbs, The People's Herbal Magazine* that was sold by members and distributed through health food shops and similar outlets. *The European Journal of Herbal Medicine* was launched in 1994 with a specific focus on herbal practice and the most recent is the *Journal of Herbal Medicine* launched in 2011, published by Elsevier with Barbara Pendry as Editor-in-Chief.

1964
100th NIMH Conference held at the Guildhall in London with presidential address given by Mr Albert Orbell FNIMH
1968
'Herbalists Triumph at Westminster – Medicines Bill Protects Freedom of Medical Choice' headline in Health from Herbs. President F Fletcher Hyde led the campaign for our ancient right to use herbal remedies.
1971
Sections 1, 2 and 3 of the British Herbal Pharmacopoeia published.
1973
NIMH launches the Education and Research Fund at Caxton Hall, Westminster, London.
1978
Hein Zeylstra established the School of Herbal Medicine in Tunbridge Wells on behalf of the NIMH Education Fund.
1990
NIMH approved herbal training clinics in Brighton, Bristol, Coventry, Exeter, London, Manchester and Winchester. NIMH Directory membership of 225.

NIMH provided clinical training for herbal students at Hydes Herbal Clinic, Leicester from1969 until Hein Zeylstra established the School of

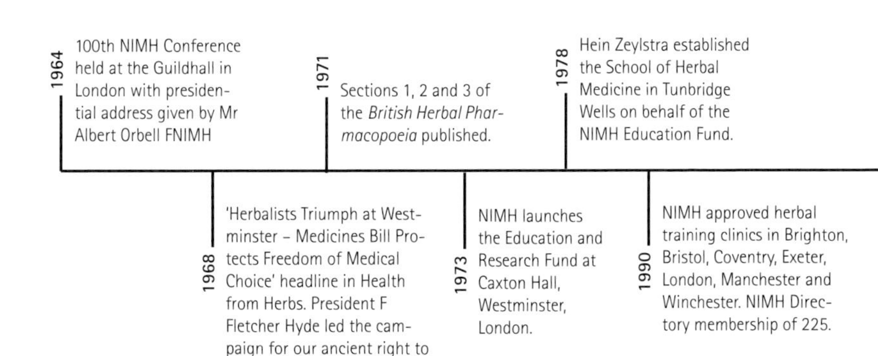

Herbal Medicine in Tunbridge Wells on behalf of the NIMH Education and Research Fund in 1978. This school later became an independent institution, known as the College of Phytotherapy and offered a full-time three year course or a four year distance learning course. These courses were transferred to the University of East London. The first full-time four year BSc (Hons) degree in herbal medicine started at Middlesex University in 1994.

The last hundred and fifty years has been a continued fight for statutory regulation of herbalists and we are all indebted to the courageous effort of Fred Fletcher Hyde when herbalists were finally recognised in the 1968 Medicines Act as being able to practise herbal medicine and prepare their own herbal medicines for patients following a one-to-one consultation. In his presidential address at the 1969 annual conference he said:

> *'We shall continue to treat each person as a unique entity and prescribe according to our judgement as to his needs. This epoch-making year will always be remembered as the year when we first obtained statutory freedom to administer the Creator's remedies to heal the sick. The future will be characterised according to the way in which you and I guard, use and extend this freedom for the benefit of humanity, under the blessing of Divine Providence'. (Fletcher Hyde 1969).*

In 1994 the UK government announced that in signing up to the main European Union Medicines Directive, it had effectively repealed Section

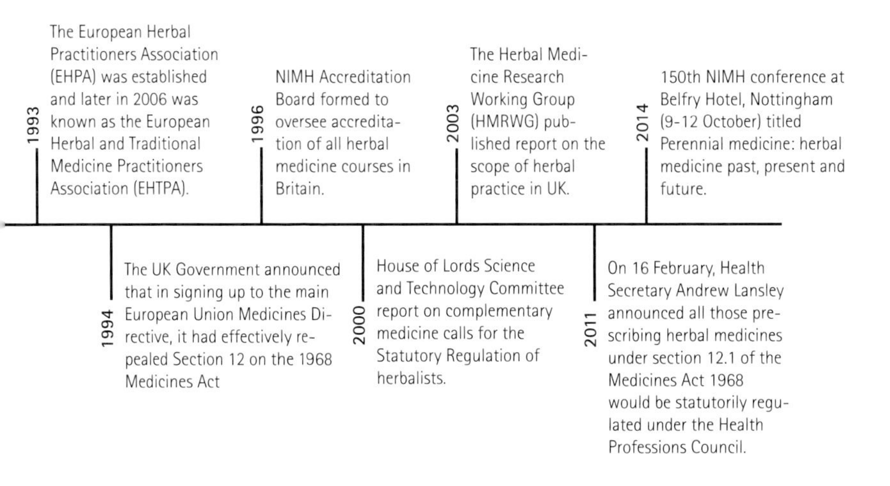
1993
The European Herbal Practitioners Association (EHPA) was established and later in 2006 was known as the European Herbal and Traditional Medicine Practitioners Association (EHTPA).
1994
The UK Government announced that in signing up to the main European Union Medicines Directive, it had effectively repealed Section 12 on the 1968 Medicines Act
1996
NIMH Accreditation Board formed to oversee accreditation of all herbal medicine courses in Britain.
2000
House of Lords Science and Technology Committee report on complementary medicine calls for the Statutory Regulation of herbalists.
2003
The Herbal Medicine Research Working Group (HMRWG) published report on the scope of herbal practice in UK.
2011
On 16 February, Health Secretary Andrew Lansley announced all those prescribing herbal medicines under section 12.1 of the Medicines Act 1968 would be statutorily regulated under the Health Professions Council.
2014
150th NIMH conference at Belfry Hotel, Nottingham (9-12 October) titled Perennial medicine: herbal medicine past, present and future.

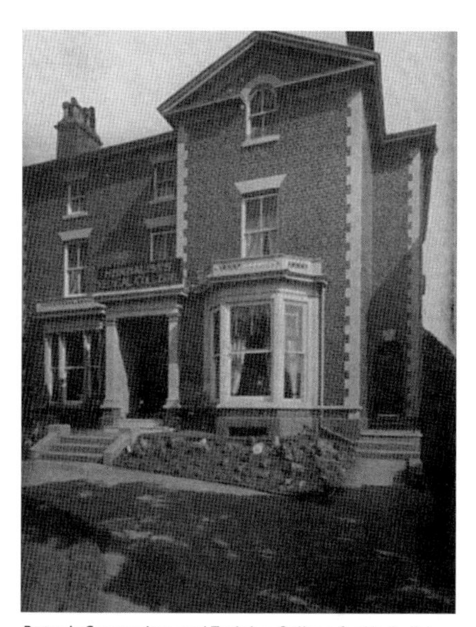

Botanic Sanatorium and Training College for Herbalists – 11 Scarisbrick Street, Southport, taken in 1902

12 of the 1968 Medicines Act. This action was reversed by a vociferous campaign in which an outraged public wrote thousands of letters in support of herbal medicine to MPs, Ministers and the Department of Health. The following years saw an increased interest in herbal medicine and in 2000, the House of Lords Select Committee report on complementary medicine called for statutory regulation of acupuncture and herbal practitioners (McIntyre 2005). The Department of Health public consultation showed an overwhelming 98 per cent opinion in favour of statutory regulation of practitioners and support of herbal medicine. The Pittilo report in 2008 set down proposed processes to bring about regulation of herbalists and finally on 16 February, 2011 Health Secretary Andrew Lansley announced in a written statement to Parliament that all those prescribing herbal medicines under Section 12.1 of the Medicines Act 1968 would be statutorily regulated under the Health Professions Council. Here three years later, we are awaiting the outcome of the recent working group convened by the government to determine whether or not herbalists should be regulated by statute.

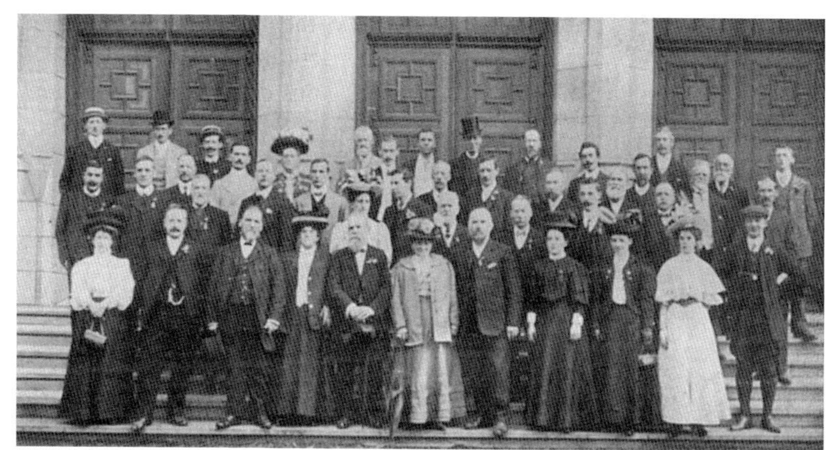

NAMH 1908 Conference Group of Members and Friends

References

Fletcher Hyde, F., 1969. Presidential address at the 1968 annual conference. *The herbal practitioner*, 18 (8), 221-227.

Jenner, A., 1964. The future of herbal medicine an address to the centenary conference. *The herbal practitioner*, 16 (1), 5-7.

MacLennan, E. and Pendry, B.A., 2011. The evolution of herbal medicine as an unorthodox branch of British medicine. The role of English legislation from antiquity to 1914. *Journal of herbal medicine*, 1 (1), 2-14.

McIntyre, M., 2005. *Herbs and herbalists: professional identity and the protection of practice. In: Reshaping herbal medicine knowledge, education and professional culture*, O'Sullivan, C., ed., London: Elsevier.

National Association of Medical Herbalists of Great Britain Ltd. *Council meeting minutes*. 21 August 1901, 27 February 1902, 25 July 1902, 4 May 1911, 2 March 1922, 15 March1923, 4 February 1948.

National Association of Medical Herbalists of Great Britain Ltd., 1908. *Year book and transactions with the directory of members for the year 1907 and 1908*. Worcester. NAMH of GB Ltd.

National Association of Medical Herbalists of Great Britain Ltd, 1908. *Jubilee souvenir year book*. Worcester: NAMH of GB Ltd.

Scientific Committee of the British Herbal Medicine Association, 1983. *British herbal pharmacopoeia*. Bournemouth: British Herbal Medicine Association.

The Tonic Prescribing Principle of 1860 in modern herbal practice

Dee Atkinson

To understand the foundations of a traditional herbal practice, we need only take a journey through the basement of Napiers at 18 Bristo Place, Edinburgh in 1990. First, we travel down a winding wooden staircase (mind your head on that light bulb) and arrive in the bowels of the building. The smell is overwhelming, a bit like burying your nose in your mother's spice cupboard on a warm day, when all the smells are in the air. There's the familiar aroma of cooking, with a sweet top note and a back note of spice, a hint of tar and something that reminds me of marmite.

Lit with harsh strip lights, it's a chaotic world down here. Wooden barrels and boxes vie for space with metal shelves, the latter groaning under the weight of dusty bags and tins. In the centre is a low table, where some glorious antique scales have been pushed to one side to make way for a shiny white plastic set, splendid in their newness. I was to learn that, twice a year, a man came down from Dundee to service those older and now relegated scales, to make sure that an ounce was, indeed, an ounce.

Turning a corner in the basement leads to the manufacturing area. Off to one side is a small room containing an enamelled set of burners, looking much bigger in the small, cramped space. Back in the main area, big 'jam' pans and massive sieves hang from hooks in the wall and row upon row of wooden shelves hold legions of liquid-filled glass jars. Old labels, written over many times, are stuck on the surface, proclaiming the contents within: blood purifier; heart tonic; composition essence No2; pruning heart...

Attached to a low, heavy table with a metal top, is a small herb press. Adapted and attached to a hydraulic press, the handle is always half down and a white bin at its side collects the liquid that drips out. To the right of this, a round metal tube with what looks like a funnel with a tap on the end, is fixed to the wall, another bucket beneath it to collect the slow drip of dark liquid. In earlier days, the edges of all the shelves would have been lined with cardboard tubs, filled with a slowly settling amber ointment.

On every surface there is action: a small wooden stool, with a drum of alcohol on it, being siphoned into a jug; scales piled high with paraffin wax for ointments; herbs being measured and weighed; and a three bar electric fire in the corner for comfort.

It is an engine room. A heart. A living history.

As we observe the scene, we are watching formulas being manufactured in the same way, and to the same recipe, as the original ones that Duncan Napier wrote in 1860. Adapted over the years by his sons, these formulas were finally pulled together and refined by his grandson, the late John Napier. John Napier was a gifted practitioner who had inherited a business and a wealth of recipes and formulas, as well as a reputation. He had also inherited over a hundred years of knowledge in how to use herbs in a specific way, in specific combinations, and with some very clear underlying principles on prescribing.

Many of the Napier formulas were multi-herb combinations, not the five to six herb blends that I had studied, but 20 to 30 herb blends, complex and interwoven. In some cases only small amounts of each active ingredient would be in the final product. These medicines were a true example of the whole being more than the sum of its individual parts. There was a synergy to each formula which I have always likened to cooking; the blends of spices mixing together in the pan to create a final, delicious dish, the meld of flavours exploding into a single unique taste.

Over the past 20 years of working with these formulas, I have coined the phrase 'The Tonic Prescribing Principle' to try to explain the ideas behind the Napiers blends. I was lucky in having access to all of the historical records and case histories as well as working for two years with someone who had been trained by John Napier.

One of Napiers' most famous formulas was The Nerve Debility Tonic. This was a complex mixture for the 'stresses and strains of modern living', for 'when one could just sit down and cry'. To quote from an early text of John Napier, 'The first action is on the nerves of digestion,

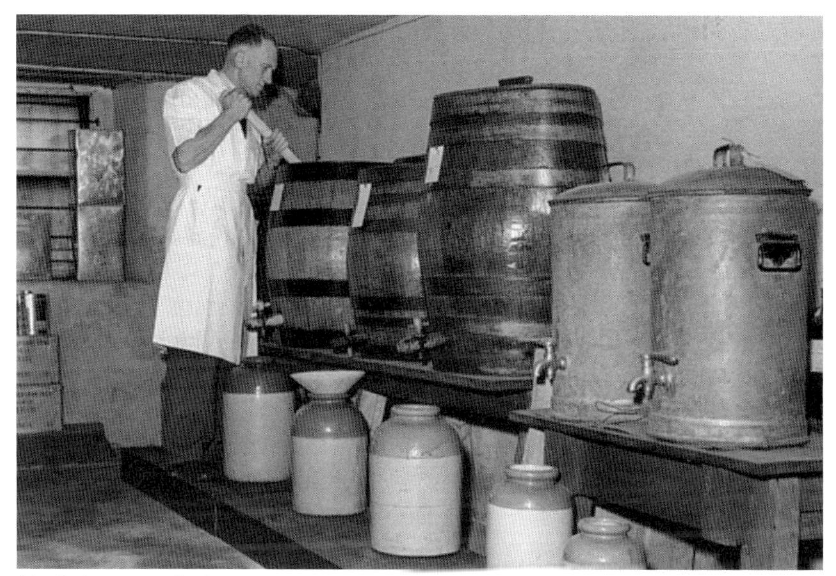

John Napier preparing tinctures

encouraging blood supply so that food may be properly digested. The nerves to the bowels are restored, easing congestion, and headaches, and blood supply to the muscles in the back and neck, to ease tension'.

It is all too easy to dismiss this explanation as being unscientific and fanciful. But behind the marketing speak of the time were some solid beliefs that had stood the test of clinical practice for over 100 years.

The Tonic Prescribing Principle is a specific way of layering a medicine to 'tone' all the body's organs. If, for example, a patient suffers from nervous anxiety and tension, the treatment was not just to use a single herb, but many herbs. In many cases, the physical presentation of anxiety touches several body systems, so we might find a combination of palpitations, headaches, constipation, sleeplessness, shortness of breath or raised blood pressure - in other words, many physical symptoms that are a result of mental anxiety. There could be physical triggers to this, for instance, overwork and underexercise are often drivers and, over the centuries, although our lives have been mechanised and improved, the basic stress drivers are often the same.

A tonic prescriber would look at all of the body systems and use herbs to support, tone and nourish these. So, blood supply would be improved, mild laxatives would support the bowels, muscle tension in neck and shoulders would be relieved and acid indigestion calmed. By toning all

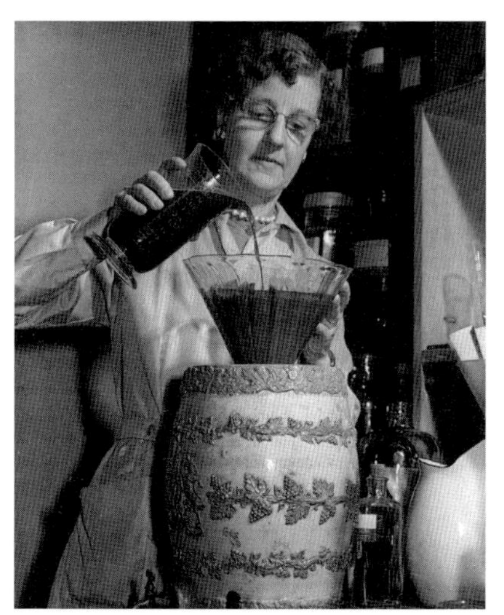

Mrs Mekkings

the body systems the whole body will gently move towards health.

All too often in medicine today we look at a single body ailment in isolation. Tension headaches are relieved by pain killers, leaving the patient constipated and with acid indigestion. The Tonic Prescribers tried to reach all organs with their prescriptions.

Napiers' Nerve Debility Tonic contained: Jamaican dogwood, saw palmetto, kola, damiana, oats, gentian, skullcap, passionflower, calamba, black cohosh, cramp bark, oregon grape, bearberry, valerian, skunk cabbage, chilli, golden seal, dandelion root, lime flowers, lobelia and marshmallow.

This complex formula, made partly by percolation of powder blends, partly by acid tinctures and partly by alcohol tinctures, is a superb example of the whole being more than the sum of the parts, as mentioned above. The main herbs in the mix are skullcap and passionflower, which work on mental anxiety and nervous stress. The skullcap was used as a tincture, a percolated fluid extract and in water infusion. The different extraction methods meant that we had something approaching whole-plant extraction.

Continuing to work through the formula, we have gentian to improve appetite and digestion, dandelion to keep the bowels regular, lime flowers to calm palpitations, black cohosh to balance hormones, saw palmetto and damiana to, again, regulate hormones as well as supporting the libido, oats to build up and restore the nervous system and bearberry for bladder health.

The thought might be that such small doses of herbs, even when fluid extracts were used, were simply not enough to have an action. But clinical experience shows otherwise. Having used this every day in my practice since 1989, I know that this combination of herbs will support the whole nervous system. It can be used for mild depression, anxiety, work-related stress, fear of flying, exam stress, and, in fact, as Mr Napier said in 1860, "for the stresses and strains of modern living".

In practice, I often combine this as an adjunct with other formulas. I may be treating menopause patients who find stress is a major issue, or I may be supporting a cancer patient who is struggling with stress. This formula is right in both situations. The low doses of each individual herb mean that we rarely see side effects; the combination simply tones and supports the system.

These complex formulas were much used by the traditional herbalists of the last century. A successful herbal practice would have built up their repertoire of formulas over many years, conversing and exchanging ideas with fellow practitioners. Napiers was no exception and letters track the course of the formulas. Exchanges with American colleagues meant new herbs were added and legislation changes caused changes in formula and name. For example, The Nerve Debility Tonic became The Herbal Tonic and eventually, in 2002, I changed the name to Skullcap, Oat and Passionflower. But, whatever the name, the formula is the same and the amazing Tonic Prescribing Principle, developed by The Napier Herbalists from 1860 onwards, is still being used in my practice today.

Yet they speak – a master class from the past

Jane Gray

The 28 May 1895 was a momentous day for herbal medicine – the National Association of Medical Herbalists (NAMH) formally signed its Memorandum and Articles of Association. Those responsible for drawing up that founding document included an article: 'to form or otherwise acquire and to maintain, extend and improve a library or libraries' that is today known as Article C.5 (NIMH, 2011, p.5). This has enabled NIMH to acquire books, research papers and other memorabilia from members bequeathing personal materials.

Why is this important? There is truth in the saying 'you can't get to where you're going unless you know where you started'. Our history shows us the path we have been walking and only with this understanding can we decide where we are heading.

Since its founding in 1864, NIMH has been supported by many hard working herbalists and sadly, only fragments of memories remain of the founding generation of herbalists. What we do know shows them to be very much men of their time and many had a high standing within their communities serving as Aldermen and Councillors. Women were often integral to the herbalists' practice collecting herbs and making up medicines, acting as nurse and receptionist, dispenser and accountant, although not represented in NIMH until the early 20th century.

As the Institute approached its 50th anniversary in 1904, a new generation of herbalists was emerging. It has been my very great privilege both as a member of NIMH Council and now as Chair of the NIMH Library Committee to be given access to the documents, libraries or practices of four notable members namely, Fred Fletcher Hyde, Thomas Bartram, Albert Priest, and here locally in Manchester, Charles Abbott.

So what did I learn from these four notable men?

Fred Fletcher Hyde (1911–2004)

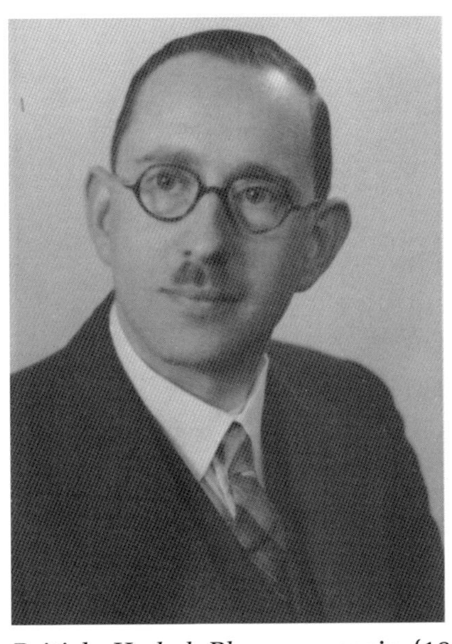

The history of Fred Fletcher Hyde's practice compiled by Serene Foster MNIMH can be found on page 39. However, late on in his life Fred bequeathed a number of herbal documents to NIMH that have been catalogued and are available to anyone visiting the library in Exeter. Much of the material Fred left to the institute relates to his herbal research of individual herbs and sets of plant illustrations. Having obtained a degree in chemistry and studied botany, Fred helped to compile the source material for two major published works: *The British Herbal Pharmacopoeia* (1983) and the *British Herbal Compendium Volume 1* (1993). Fred recognised that we needed a more scientific basis to our herbal practice and with his unique skills he was able to provide this research on behalf of the herbal medicine profession.

Fred strongly believed people should have the right of choice for herbal medicine and worked hard to defend herbal medicine as a recognised option for personal health. That we are able to use comfrey in modern practice may well be down to the work of this one man. Fred entered into correspondence with authorities including the World Health Organisation and compiled safety data on comfrey that prevented an outright ban on this herb.

There were many at the time, who opposed herbal medicine yet Fred quietly but firmly defended both herbalists as practitioners and the public's right of choice. Fred worked with a number of Government departments and working parties seeking to preserve the integrity of herbal medicine and medical herbalists. In addition to lobbying politically for herbal medicine Fred also devoted much time to the professional body and served as President of NIMH for 8 years (1968-1975) and for a further 30 years, he was Director of Research.

Thomas Bartram (1912–2009)

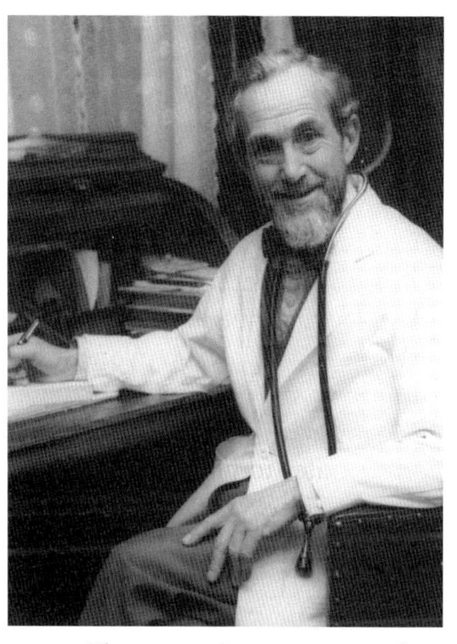

Thomas was a practising medical herbalist for 35 years, working from his home in Boscombe near Bournemouth. Thomas also trained as a homeopath and used this knowledge in his practice alongside that of herbal medicine. Through wide-ranging and extensive reading he absorbed an understanding of many naturopathic treatments that he incorporated into his herbal practice. A deeply spiritual man in the widest sense of the word Thomas founded *Grace Magazine* in 1960 which he continued to publish and edit for a further 49 years. The magazine encouraged readers to have a wider view of health than simply that of the body.

Having had a hospital career before becoming a herbalist Thomas truly valued the difference herbal medicine could make to his patients' health. He was not content to simply give medicine to those who consulted him, but having a strong belief that herbs could make an important contribution to the health of the nation he founded a herbal medicine company. Named after the famous herbalist and botanist John Gerard (c1545-1612), his company Gerard House, manufactured and sold a range of herbal medicines based on successful formulae that Thomas had used in his own practice.

Herbal medicine was more than just an interest or a job, it was a passion, and his wish to educate others into the benefits of herbal medicine led to Thomas spending 10 years of his life compiling research and producing the famous *Encyclopaedia of Herbal Medicine* (1995). All his research files are now in the NIMH library, many annotated with notes and comments in his own hand. Right up until a month before his death at the age of 96 he was still working on another compilation – as his son Roger said, "he was dedicated to his vision". Thomas Bartram also found the time to serve his professional body as a council member of the National Institute of Medical Herbalists for a number of years.

Albert Priest (c.1920–2001)

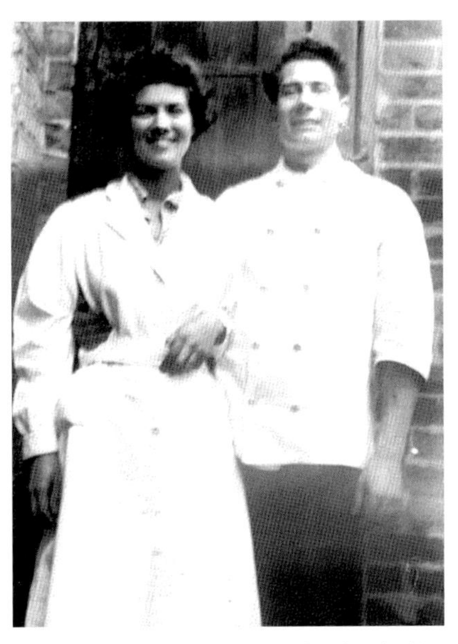

Albert set up his practice as a medical herbalist on the Talgarth Road, London in 1948. In common with many herbalists of the time, Albert Priest lived in the upper part of the house with his wife and two daughters whilst the lower part was converted into a consulting room and waiting room. In the basement he stored his herbs and made up and dispensed herbal medicines. In many ways Albert couldn't have picked a worse time to start his career as a herbalist. The National Health Service was born in 1948 and the public adopted it enthusiastically. The challenge for herbalists was how to make a living at a time when orthodox healthcare was free and seemed to offer, through advances in surgery and medicine, the route to better health for the whole country. In speaking of these times, his daughter Kate said, "he just kept going because his patients kept getting better".

Albert Priest was not a man to rest on his laurels and became a life-long learner. On visiting his extensive library in Talgarth Road, I found sections of books on conventional medicine including operating theatre techniques, anatomy, physiology, conventional drugs and also books on other complementary therapies. Albert developed an interest in iridology and even taught himself German in order to translate Theodor Kriege's books into English. Being willing to learn from both the past as well as contemporary research he also studied medical astrology and trained as an osteopath and naturopath.

Albert operated a loans service for those books in his library which he felt would be useful for patients to read. He made cards out for chosen titles and marked with the patient's name and date, allowed the patient to take books as part of their treatment.

Albert also developed a collection of physical and mental health exercises which he compiled onto a series of numbered cards. The exercises were designed to cover all skeletal and anatomical health problems and relevant cards were issued to patients alongside their herbal prescription. One which caught my eye – obviously designed to help improved digestion went as follows:

> *'Decide that for one week you will chew every mouthful of food at least 50 times. If you realise that unconsciously you have swallowed a mouthful without doing so, stop the meal immediately and take no more food until the next meal.'*

Another instruction which was probably aimed at improving posture and circulation read:

> *'Decide that for one week you will not cross the legs one over the other on sitting down. If you do so, give yourself a vigorous pinch on the fleshy part of the inner thigh.'*

He used these tools as he felt appropriate, integrating them into individual treatment plans for his patients.

Albert drew extensively on the knowledge of his wife Lillian who had trained as a homeopath and often referred patients to her for part of their treatment. Albert and Lilian were very much a team shown by their collaboration in producing *Herbal Medication – a Clinical and Dispensary Handbook* (1983). In fact the whole family were involved in the practice. Kate recalls going out with her father identifying and collecting plants for him to make into medicines. As a teenager she worked in the dispensary making up many of her father's formulas like his own 'Mist tuss' – a liquid coltsfoot compound which she remembers being given to her regularly as a child whenever she had a cough.

Mr Priest conducted his clinical training with Albert Orbell – himself a FNIMH and past President of NIMH. The example set by Mr. Orbell greatly influenced Albert and once qualified, he too became involved with the professional association. Albert's personal interest in continuing education was fulfilled as Editor of the NIMH journal, *Herbal Practitioner* for 20 years and as Director of Education. In this capacity, Albert wrote a set of units for use by herbal medicine students. A complete set of these is available in the NIMH library. Amazingly, Albert also found time to serve as the Vice Dean of the British College of Naturopathy and Osteopathy.

Charles Abbott (1889–1983)

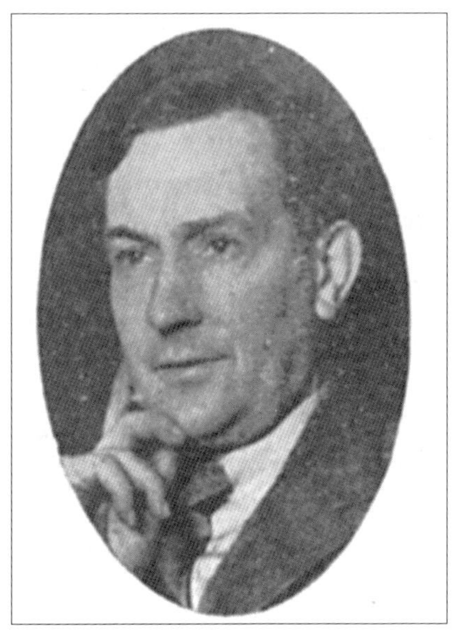

Charles though of a similar generation to the other three gentlemen was very different and a larger than life character. Brought up in the mining community of Leigh, near Manchester as a child, Charles knew real poverty first hand. His first full time job was at the age of 12, as a messenger boy at the mines and a year later, he became a miner because the wage was better.

However, some five years later, Charles experienced a personal health crisis when he was diagnosed with tuberculosis. Given the conditions in the mines at the time and before the advent of antibiotics, all four doctors Charles consulted had nothing to offer. Charles went to see a herbalist and had a life changing experience. His tuberculosis was treated successfully with dietary advice and herbal medicine. This sparked Charles' interest in herbal medicine and he studied as much as he could whilst still working in the mines. Three years later aged 20, Charles passed the entry examinations and became a member of NAMH.

Charles ran his public clinic on Railway Road, which was also his home for some of the early years, in the centre of Leigh. There he treated the ordinary working class members of the community including miners and their families. In those communities time off work meant no money coming in and families suffered so Charles focused on getting people better – fast. For wealthier patients, Charles maintained a private consulting room at his home in a better part of the town – I did wonder if, unknowingly, these privileged patients subsidised the work he did at Railway Road?

For a short while I was privileged to work as locum in Railway Road, and there met Peter Berry. Peter had initially worked for Charles Abbott as a boy and in later life he returned, with his wife, Jean, to work at the practice. Jean became the dispenser and Peter made up the special medicine combinations and mixtures that Charles had developed over the years. These ranged from Nasal Drops, Eye Drops, various ointments and creams and a collection of specialist mixtures including Anti-Spas (used as a topical rub for neuralgic pain as well as a systemic in asthma mixtures) and Neuro Co (to help reduce stress and anxiety). One formula I was especially fascinated by was Sure Cure. Peter told me that this mix had been formulated by Charles as a treatment for Spanish flu which devastated much of the world following World War One.

Charles Abbott was very protective of his formulations and designed them in a complex and interconnected way which meant that no one could know the exact composition of each mixture. For example, Sure Cure contained a percentage of coltsfoot compound, which in turn contained a proportion of Anti-Spas mix but without having all the recipes you could not know the exact amount of each plant used in the mixture.

Charles was fiercely independent, with a deep conviction that what he was doing was right. This in turn gave him the courage to tackle any adversaries face on and he was challenged by doctors and coroners in the courts several times with accusations of causing death by malpractice. Charles took on each accusation in public and won on all accounts. Subsequently, he wrote up some of these matters and published a book to sell to his patients and members of the public informing them of 'the truth'. One example is *Rex v Charles Clement Abbott a Transcript* (1922) published from shorthand notes of his trial, a copy of which is in the NIMH library. One quote from his robust defence of the physio-medical concept of treating disease with botanic medicines states:

> *'One would have thought the time had arrived when all schools of thought could be utilised to combat the diseases which take annual toll of thousands of lives in this country, but instead of that the allopaths have arrogated to themselves the right to condemn all other schools of healing. Why should an allopathic doctor be called (as in this trial) to prove that another school of healing, of which he is ignorant, is entirely wrong. There is neither logic nor justice in the affair'.*

Charles' patients however trusted him implicitly and his practice continued to flourish. Whilst working there as locum I saw some elderly patients who had fond memories of Mr Abbott saying, "you didn't tell Mr Abbott where your pain was – he told you". Peter recalls seeing the waiting room completely full with patients queuing out of the surgery and into Railway Road. Perhaps reflecting the poverty that Charles experienced in his childhood, it was interesting to learn from Peter that Charles never forgot his mining roots. These accounts show people continue to remember Mr Abbot with admiration, deep respect and a tinge of awe.

Charles Abbott worked hard to defend the public's right to choose herbal medicine and all his life tried to educate to that effect. He joined NIMH and wrote articles for the early journals sharing his expertise on the effects of diet on health – he was a strong believer that you could not expect health to grow from an unhealthy diet. The last medical herbalist to work at Charles Abbott's practice in Railway Road was Zoe Naylor who is currently compiling a more extensive history about Charles and his herbal practice.

Past Masters

Having been privileged to 'meet' these herbalists in various ways through their patients, their writings, their prescriptions and their families I began to see some of the traits they shared. Living in the communities they served, many of them worked from home. This meant that they were in one sense inviting patients to be part of 'their' family. They were an integral part of the community providing a healthcare service.

Interestingly many of the founder members of NIMH were Non-Conformist, teetotallers with strong moral objections to alcohol. This meant that they did not, as most of us do today, use alcoholic tinctures. Their training enabled them to make their own water extracts and formulate their own prescriptions, often making stock bottles of favourite combinations.

They were pragmatic, not afraid to combine skills, often working with massage, osteopathy, homeopathy, iridology and other modalities. Whatever would work to achieve maximum benefit for their patients – a truly holistic approach. All of them held a strong belief in the benefit of herbal medicine and defended the right of the public to choose herbal medicine. They believed herbal medicine had a professional future and they were not afraid to publicise their viewpoints.

All four herbalists continued right up to the end of their lives treating patients, learning and extending their personal boundaries. They were widely read and continued to be interested in new approaches and ideas. All engendered deep respect from their patients and herbal medicine was an integral part of their life – it defined them. It doesn't mean that they didn't have other interests – all married and had families but their overwhelming interest was herbal medicine. For them herbal medicine was a way of life and a vocation. Speaking for myself, their path is one I am happy to continue walking in the 21st century.

References

Abbott, C.C., 1934. *Rex V. Charles Clement Abbot, Wednesday March 29th 1933. Transcript of shorthand note (being the full account of the trial of C.C. Abbott for manslaughter).* England: Charles Clement Abbott.

Bartram, T., 1995. *Bartrams' encyclopaedia of herbal medicine.* London: Robinson Publishing.

Bradley, P.R., ed., 1993. *British herbal compendium: volume 1: a handbook of scientific information on widely used plant drugs.* Bournemouth: The British Herbal Medicine Association.

Priest, A.W. and Priest, L.R., 1983. *Herbal medication a clinical and dispensary handbook.* Essex: C.W. Daniel Company.

National Institute of Medical Herbalists, 2011. *Memorandum and Articles of Association.* [online]. Available from: http://www.nimh.org.uk/wp-content/titkosuploads/2012/03/Mems-Arts-Byelaws-Nov-111.pdf [Accessed 02 May 2014].

Scientific Committee of the British Herbal Medicine Association, 1983. *British herbal pharmacopoeia.* Bournemouth: The British Herbal Medicine Association.

Herbal practice in London's East End between the Wars, and the founding of the Hospital for Natural Healing

Kevin Orbell-McSean

The following is a glimpse into the world of organised herbal medicine between the wars, seen through the eyes of the late Albert Orbell FNIMH, a medical herbalist who practised in the East End of London, along with an account of the founding of the Hospital For Natural Healing (HNH). Albert was a founding member and Life Governor of the HNH, and President of the National Institute of Medical Herbalists (NIMH) from 1963–65.

The story is adapted from Albert Orbell's professional memoir, and the Annual Reports of the HNH, which are an inspiration to read. Additional information has been obtained from the former in-house NIMH magazine 'Health from Herbs – a journal of organic medicine', and Albert's obituary to which Mr. Albert Priest FNIMH made a significant contribution. The whole account is bolstered by personal memory of much time shared with my grandfather, Albert Orbell, asking questions about herbal medicine, helping out in his pharmacy and listening to many tales of herbal practice in times gone by.

Albert Orbell's early interest in medicine had a strictly orthodox perspective as he studied hard, nurturing an ambition to follow in the wake of the great surgeons of the day whom he assisted in the operating theatres of the London Hospital. Unfortunately his surgical ambitions were thwarted by a severe bout of rheumatic fever, following an intensive period in theatre treating overwhelming numbers of allied casualties from the German spring offensive of Easter 1917. As a result of his illness the young Albert was left with a bad chorea, and the uncontrollable tremor put an end to any surgical ambitions.

One day, during his convalescence, Albert was running some photographic experiments in his darkroom and splashed some chemicals on his coat. His brother George, having lost an arm, had recently returned wounded from the trenches, (he was awarded the Distinguished Conduct Medal and Bar) and suggested Albert go to Charlie Gapp's herb shop in Bethnal Green to buy some quilla bark, the infusion of which is an excellent fabric cleaner and conditioner. Charlie Gapp was a herbalist of some repute, and when Albert presented himself Charlie took one look at Albert's chorea and told him that he'd be better off buying some mistletoe for his nerves, than quilla bark for his coat. Albert was pointedly uninterested, and just bought his threepence worth of quilla bark. The quilla bark did an astonishingly good job on his coat, and Albert realised there might be something to herbs after all.

A couple of days later (too ashamed to return to Charlie Gapp after dismissing his offer of help) Albert bought one ounce of fine-cut mistletoe from a herbalist in Angel Lane, Stratford, E15. Making up the dried herb into a traditional ounce-to-the-pint decoction, Albert took a wineglassful three times a day. Over three weeks the symptoms cleared up, much to the chagrin of Albert's doctor who threw him out of his surgery and told him never to return, on account of Albert's resorting to 'quack remedies'. From this point on Albert devoted his life to the study and practice of herbal medicine, avidly reading the works of the leading medical herbalists, Coffin, Skelton, Thurston, Beach, Cook and others, discovering a system of natural medicine that came as nothing short of a revelation.

As Albert's knowledge increased he had to walk miles in search of herbal shops that stocked some of the more obscure herbs he needed to treat his friends and family. Herbal shops were mostly to be found in the backstreets of the poorer districts of London's East End, although they were not uncommon in north and south London as well.

In those days relatively few herbalists were members of the National Association of Medical Herbalists (NAMH), the only professional body of herbalists at the time, and fewer still had consulting rooms, with the quiet end of the herbal shop counter being used to consult with patients.

Most herbalists' shops sold proprietary medicines as well as herbs, and some an even more diversified stock.

One herbalist's shop was more akin to an oil shop, selling items such as candles, matches, gas mantles and paraffin oil for heaters, as well as two or three pence worth of cough mixture, or whatever other herbal remedy the customer required. He had a good reputation as a herbalist despite his eclectic stock, with many impressive cures to his name.

One day, in a side street of Canning Town, Albert had the good fortune to discover 'The Little Herb Shop'. Confronted by an elderly gentleman in shirtsleeves, stiff starched cuffs turned back and sporting two pairs of iron-rimmed glasses, Albert was initially put off by Mr. J. C. Purdue's brusque manner: "Well, what do you want? Come along, come along boy, I haven't all day to waste". But when Albert asked if he had the unusual herb he was looking for Mr. Purdue replied, "Of course – you name the herb and I've got it, and if not I'll soon get it". Meeting the proprietor, who was also a member of NAMH, proved to be the turning point in Albert's herbal medicine career.

From that day on Mr. Purdue became Albert's greatest friend and teacher. Mr. Purdue was a remarkable man, loved by rich and poor alike. It is no exaggeration to say that thousands owed him their life, and many he treated without payment, although he himself was not a rich man. To all intent and purposes, Albert served an old fashioned apprenticeship, studying in his spare time whilst learning the profession first hand from a man whose years of experience stretched back into the Victorian era. This is how he got started.

One morning a letter arrived from Mr. Purdue, a five-shilling postal order enclosed, telling Albert to have a good breakfast and to come at once. By the dim light of a gas mantle in what was once a kitchen, Albert's heart sank when he was shown a mountain of bottles, all shapes and sizes, stacked in wooden boxes. Given precise instructions on how to clean the bottles, he rolled up his sleeves and set to work. To his surprise he enjoyed the work, which passed Mr. Purdue's inspection of placing selected bottles against a sheet of white paper, the best way to spot a stain.

Albert was soon making up herbal preparations including Smoking Mixture, passing rose petals, lavender flowers, coltsfoot leaves and more through a large wire sieve, looking quite the apprentice by the end of the day, covered from head to toe in white coltsfoot dander. From there it was on to making pill-mass and rolling pills of different formulations, making batches of twelve different ointments as well as liniments, cough mixtures and a thousand-and-one other little jobs that could only be learned from experience, but not always without incident.

People today would be surprised to learn that effective herbal antibiotic therapy preceded Alexander Fleming's discovery of penicillin by many decades. One day, after the young apprentice's particularly thorough cleaning of the large, long stockroom at the top of the shop, Mr. Purdue was upset to discover the enamel pot of mouldy ointment had been scoured spotless: "Do you realise it took me four weeks to grow that mould? It's peculiar to that particular ointment, and essential to curing barber's rash," (sycosis barbae, a chronic and recalcitrant folliculitis). Mr. Purdue's ointment was found to perform what seemed like miracles before the antibiotic era, curing many obstinate skin rashes.

Cough mixture was another medicine with an 'antibiotic' element. Using glycerine, block juice of liquorice was rendered to a liquid in an enamel pot and sterile gauze strips were laid over the surface. This was allowed to stand for a few weeks until the surface was covered with a reasonably thick bloom of mould, when the gauze strips were carefully lifted away in one piece taking away all of the mould. The liquorice was then described as 'penicilliated'. Although still very good without the mould treatment (which is how I make it today) the cough mixture was certainly more effective for bronchitis when made with the mould treatment. There was no doubting Mr Purdue had a wonderful pharmacy, and the skill to match it.

When serving behind the counter there were many things to get used to, not least the customers. Albert's first customer wanted "three penn'orth orange peel" which he couldn't find anywhere, until Mr. Purdue said, "Dear oh dear. She means orange pills, twelve for threepence". Then there was the cockney slang, "Animated Pictures of Queen Anne for my cold", meaning ammoniated tincture of quinine, or "Hippy Hippy Hacky Wine to make my baby sick", which meant ipecacuanha wine, a preparation of the dried and powdered liquid extract of ipecacuanha root added to sherry. There was never a dull moment, with shifty looking fellows coming in from the docks, trying to sell black market goods and contraband.

Before the Second World War and the birth of the welfare state, poor people lived in truly deprived circumstances. Even for the urban poor who were working, it was not unusual to have to pawn essentials such as the bedclothes or kitchenware on a Monday morning, redeeming them on a Friday evening after being paid - the 1920s version of a payday loan. For ordinary working people trying to survive on such tight budgets, herbal medicine was, of necessity if not preference, the first recourse when illness struck. As a result, herbalists could expect to see the full spectrum of disease presenting in their practice, and might also carry out minor surgery like snaring nasal polyps and stitching wounds, if they felt able and had the instruments.

Albert learnt a wealth of knowledge from Mr. Purdue, including how to recognise and treat a myriad of different diseases from the cases that came through the door of the Little Herb Shop. One day a mother brought in a child covered with a particular type of rash. She had just come from the doctor who had dismissed the case as something the child had eaten, but the mother wasn't happy with all the angry little spots. Albert didn't recognise the symptoms and called Mr. Purdue to have a look, who with some alarm and no hesitation, diagnosed smallpox and told the woman to find another doctor immediately.

Years later during a smallpox epidemic in West Ham, Albert was called to see many such cases, though he had to refer them to the medical authorities as required by law, receiving a letter of acknowledgement from the Borough Medical Officer and a small remuneration for each case. Despite frequent contact and no inoculation, Albert never caught smallpox himself, nor did his family or other members of households he was called to with a smallpox case. He attributed this to the powerful prophylactic effect of *Sarracenia purpurea* L. (purple pitcher plant), a North American herb which he prescribed for people in contact with sufferers.

Shortly after Mr. Purdue died Albert joined the London Branch of NAMH and established his own practice. His surgery was a busy practice and opened at nine-thirty in the morning, when there could be people queuing down the street and round the corner. It was often past eleven at night by the time he saw the last patient, fitting in a list of house calls between morning and evening surgery. This remained the case for decades. On a busy day Albert's devoted wife Lilian was known to mix well over a hundred bottles of medicine in the course of a day's work, besides being a mother and running the home.

There were herb gathering forays to Epping Forest, Wanstead flats, Canvey Island and other localities, wildcrafting herbs to stock Albert's pharmacy, Mr. Purdue style. He mostly used fluid extracts rather than tinctures, and made several varieties of pills and ointments, lotions and liniments, as well as different stock mixtures to form a base for treating the more common ailments.

Almost all of Albert's time was taken up with activities related to herbal medicine. It was no wonder that, aged around eleven when I first expressed a serious interest in taking up the profession, Albert said, "Well my boy, there's no finer work in the world, but be sure of one thing, you will have to marry your profession as well as your wife."

House calls were usually for patients who were too sick to come to the surgery. One such case, typical of many, was to a little girl of eighteen months suffering from pneumonia. The doctor had tried everything to no avail, and that morning had told the distraught mother that her daughter had only hours left to live, saying he would drop round with the death certificate the next morning.

When Albert called, the child's respiration was shallow and rapid, her head occasionally tossing from side to side in search of oxygen, lips encrusted with sores and fingers picking and clutching at the bedclothes. The only hope lay in giving her a lobelia emetic to force a sudden diaphragmatic contraction against the base of the lungs, expelling the infected mucous which was choking her respiratory system. With some difficulty, infusions of elderflower, peppermint and lobelia were separately administered in a particular sequence, about a quarter of a teacup in total. Approximately three minutes later the child convulsed, vomiting up a quantity of brown phlegm. This happened three times, after which the exhausted child slept. Her breathing sounded a little better, and Albert told the mother he thought the child would recover. When he called again that evening, the little girl's breathing was much improved. The doctor returned next morning, death certificate already made out, to find the little girl propped up with pillows in bed, taking a little warm milk. The doctor tore up the death certificate saying that a miracle had occurred, unaware that the miracle was due to the skilful intervention of a medical herbalist who had administered a lobelia emetic.

There are instances mentioned in Albert's memoir of how either he, or the patient's family writing under his direction, wrote to the Minister of Health stating the facts of a case, asking the Minister for his authority to continue giving herbal treatment in controversial cases where orthodox practitioners were insisting only they should treat the patient. Replies were always received in a day or two, and in each case Albert's right to continue treatment was sanctioned, despite being an unregistered practitioner. I'm not sure which seems stranger in this day and age

– the speedy reply or the right to treat, granted by a politician, in preference to established orthodox medicine!

Some patients simply couldn't afford treatment, though their need was undeniable, in which case the compassionate practitioner gave either heavily discounted or free treatment. As well as Albert, there were several other kind and principled practitioners in the area including Mr. Willis of Stratford, Mr. Smith of Plaistow and Mr. Dawes of Forest Gate. This was all very well, but such practitioners were not wealthy men, giving their services at a reasonable price to start with. For instance, Albert didn't charge a consultation fee, not even for house calls.

Albert approached some kindly patients and a committee was formed, the objective being to found an association of lay people who were interested in herbal medicine, with the result that in the early 1930s the Association for Natural Healing (ANH), was established. The name was registered at Somerset House as a charity, and a Chairman, Secretary and Treasurer were elected. In just a couple of years the membership of the ANH grew to more than two hundred. The membership fee was two shillings (10p) a year, and dances, outings and educational meetings on health and a variety of subjects were held at least every month.

The ANH country rambles were particularly popular, often in Epping Forest or Wanstead Flats, invariably having an optional herb gathering/identification theme, with prizes for the top three people who had gathered the most varied specimens, and could name them. The country rambles and seaside trips were organised very much with children in mind, fresh air and healthy exercise being just the antidote for young people growing up in the smog, grime and poverty of London's East End. The selfless desire of ANH members to help their fellows, with their great enthusiasm, dedication and hard work, was the most impressive and heart-warming tribute of goodwill to humanity.

As soon as ANH funds permitted, patients unable to pay for their herbal treatment were given a letter of recommendation, signed by two ANH members, entitling them to four weeks herbal treatment. The practitioner was paid four shillings (20p) and although initially it didn't cover the cost, compassionate practitioners no longer had to give generous concessions at their own expense. There was one condition - subsidised patients were asked to join the ANH. Not obligatory, and the membership fee did not have to be paid all at once, as little as tuppence (1p) a week was acceptable. In time, other practitioners were invited to join the scheme, with Bob Willis and Horace Smith, members of the NAMH, among the first to sign up.

The ANH went from strength to strength, and inspired by the enthusiasm of the members who wanted nothing less than to establish a hospital for herbal medicine, Albert Orbell and Horace Smith organised a committee with other idealists who had a sincere wish to help humanity. They resolved to find premises for a clinic where people could have access to any form of nature-cure treatment, regardless of the means to pay.

Ambitious as they were, that was just the short-term plan. The long-term aim was to have an in-patient facility, a full-blown natural therapy hospital, and a teaching faculty for training practitioners - and not just herbalists - to be called The School of Reform Medicine. The committee members wanted to establish a true home for natural healing, with standards that would make it impossible for the authorities to ignore the immense benefits and potential of the natural medicine approach to health care.

These altruistic idealists put their hands in their own pockets to provide the initial funding, and not long after, in 1935, a house was rented at 237 Romford Road, Forest Gate, London E7. Donations started to come in from the most unlikely sources. The committee was re-christened The Governing Board, and after much negotiating correspondence with the Minister of Health, they were permitted to call the clinic The Hospital for Natural Healing. Meanwhile, the members of the ANH pledged their funds and future efforts to the establishment and operation of the hospital.

In the first year, the Hospital for Natural Healing treated four hundred and forty-five patients over the course of two thousand three hundred and ninety-seven consultations. Ten percent of the patients were officially discharged cured with a further ten percent given an unofficial discharge. (A period of observation, appropriate to the disease, was required for an official discharge, but once they were better, human nature being what it is, not all patients were inclined to attend for further consultations). Ten patients were referred to other institutions as they were either too ill for outpatient treatment, or required surgery. When considering the relatively small percentage discharged cured, it must be remembered that the vast majority of cases had been given up as hopeless and incurable by the orthodox profession, and many others sought relief from ongoing degenerative disease from which it would be difficult to ever be pronounce 'cured'.

All this activity was funded by donations and patients' payments, with a small amount coming from collection boxes. In that first year, the total costs for running the hospital came to £527, 10s 9d.

It is interesting to note that at this time West Ham Borough Council was very supportive of professional herbal medicine and the endeavour of the Governing Board to make herbal medicine readily available to its residents, declaring the work of the hospital a social service and offering such help as they were able to give. The five herbal practitioners at the hospital worked voluntarily about a half day a week in their special areas of interest. Albert Orbell treated heart, lung and rheumatic disease, Horace Smith focussed on general practice and children's ailments, and Bob Willis cardiac, GIT, skin and blood disease. Mr. Wheeler's interest was skin and hair conditions and Ronald Leisk mental and nervous disease and osteopathic treatment. The hospital's own independent Lady Almoner's department adjusted the cost of treatment to suit the convenience of patients with limited means.

The hospital was pervaded with a heartfelt sense of goodwill and love for humanity, patients and staff alike, which comes across very clearly in the hospital's Annual Reports. One returning patient was heard to say to a new patient, "Even the saddest souls which enter here, smile before they leave," saying much about the ethos of the Hospital for Natural Healing, and I suspect for many herbal practices today.

During the third year of operation (1937-1938) new and larger premises had been found, not far away in Sprowston Road, and a nurse and pharmacist were taken on, (the only salaried personnel). The Governing Board's plans for the School of Reform Medicine were well advanced; the curriculum was endorsed by the Headmasters Association and accepted by the Principle of West Ham Technical College, who pledged all necessary resources to teach the pre-medical subjects. For the first time herbal medicine was ready to enter the mainstream education system.

The School of Reform Medicine was all set to achieve its potential when the Second World War broke out, and to the deep regret of the Governing Board, the activities of the school had to be postponed indefinitely. Other ambitions were thwarted too. The x-ray machine fund (close to realisation), the building extension fund and all activities other than the core business of seeing patients, had to be shelved. Even the clinic had to close for a month while the building was made ready for air raids, the windows sandbagged, an air-raid shelter constructed for

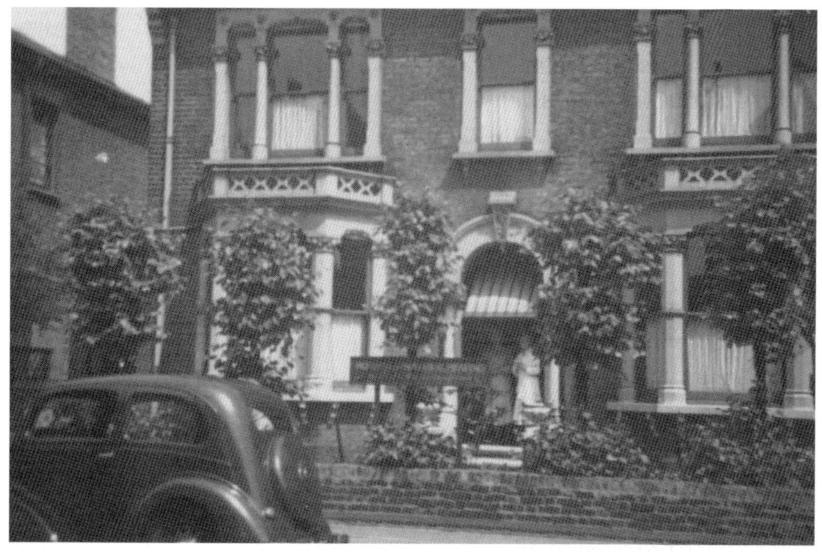

Hospital for Natural Healing, Sprowston Road, London E15, 1950s

the patients and the more valuable medicinal extracts and other medicaments moved to a safe place.

The Second World War brought mixed blessings for the herbal profession. Many of the raw materials used in a herbal pharmacy were in short supply, or simply unavailable. There was a staff shortage. The hospital's State Registered Nurse, pharmacist, and some practitioners were reassigned or volunteered for war work.

You might arrive at your surgery in the morning to find it bombed out. Albert's surgery suffered air-raid damage a couple of times, before it was finally bombed flat. A terrible blow, but he carried on by doing house calls helped by cousin Don, his best friend and right-hand-man, who converted Albert's Ford 8 car into a mobile herbal pharmacy. Medicines were dispensed parked by the kerb outside the patient's house, the sound of bombing raids frequently providing the backdrop as Albert and Don went about the work of herbal practice. By evening's end, on occasion, they found themselves weaving around fresh bomb craters through the blackout, bombed gas mains shooting up plumes of fire, water mains gushing, rubble everywhere. Such was the life of a medical herbalist in wartime.

Doctors were in short supply too, so the work of herbal practitioners provided an acknowledged important contribution to the war effort. Albert was allowed extra petrol rations to facilitate herb forays to the countryside; local hospitals would take his referrals for treatment, including surgery; sickness certificates were accepted from qualified herbalists.

On more than one occasion an officer appeared at the door of the Hospital for Natural Healing, looking for soldiers whose case might be doubtful, but in every instance accepted the certification of the practitioner in charge. Practitioners at the hospital could prescribe extra milk rations for special cases. Extra tea and sugar rations were provided to allow for patients' needs. The HNH was indeed given every consideration by official departments, for the work they were doing.

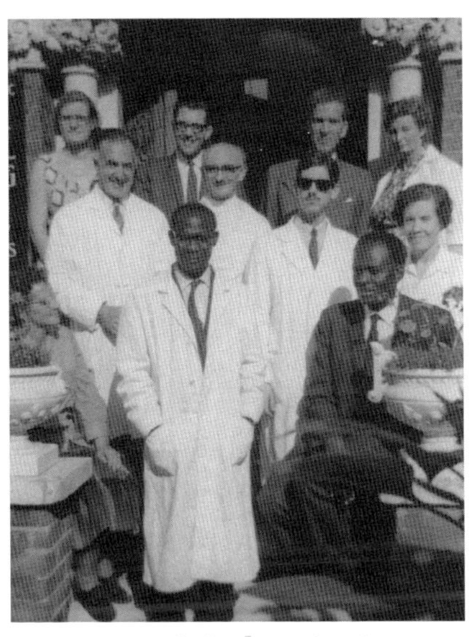

Hospital for Natural Healing, Student Group late 1950s

In the post-war years it was often a bigger job to keep the doors of the hospital open than it had been during the war. Funds were hard to come by, the lease on the building was about to expire and the prospect of its renewal seemed hopeless. People everywhere were tired of struggling, tired of sacrifice. Who could blame them? But the Governing Board, who had been through hard times before, were not ready to quit.

Appeals were made for help. Gifts of money were received, and some practitioners in the North of England, too far away to give service, sent medicine bottles, fluid extracts, pills, instruments and many other items so essential in running the hospital. The National Institute of Medical Herbalists dipped deeply into its reserves on more than one occasion to help out. In 1947, eclectic up to this time, the hospital declared itself fundamentally herbal, aligning its activities much more closely with the National Institute of Medical Herbalists and the education programme was revived.

In 1958 NIMH decided to dispose of its head office in Thundersley, Essex, and purchased the Hospital for Natural Healing's building in Sprowston Road, and didn't ask any rent from the Governing Board. About the same time a grateful patient, who had come from Switzerland especially for treatment, made a substantial cash donation to the

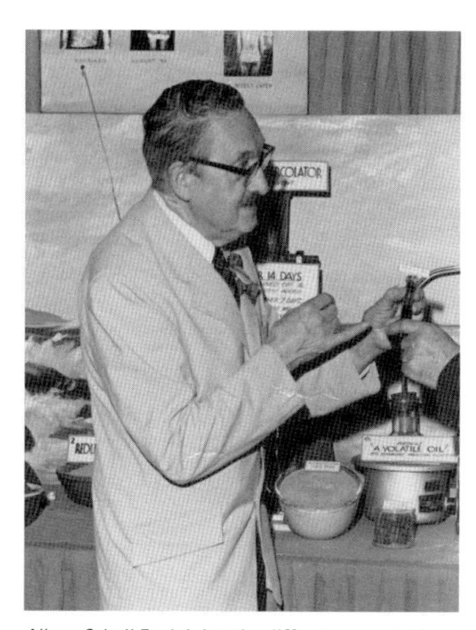
Albert Orbell Explaining the different preparations of Fucus vesiculosis (at a NIMH Conference) c1970

hospital. Between these two events the hospital was back on a sound footing, and could plan for the future. The HNH became the education centre for training future NIMH members. Indeed, my own memory of first contact with NIMH was as a lad of seven or eight in the late 1950s, being a pathology model for students taking their final clinical exam.

The 1960s and early 1970s saw a hiatus in the numbers of new practitioners coming through, likely due, among other reasons, to the introduction of the National Health Service and the threat posed to professional herbal medicine in the years before the 1968 Medicine's Act, which did not bode well for people considering a career in herbal medicine. By the mid 1970s the stalwart practitioners of the Clinic for Natural Healing (as it was now called) were ageing and retiring, with no new practitioners to carry on the work. No longer possible to continue, the Governing Board made an appeal to NIMH who had recently established, through the Charity Commission, an Educational Trust Fund. The object, in accordance with the terms of the clinic's charitable charter, was to found a centre where a school establishing the heart of herbal medicine in all its aspects could be located. The NIMH Educational Trust Fund and the Governing Board of the Clinic for Natural Healing worked together to achieve this amalgamation, with Albert Orbell becoming one of the trustees. Although that marked the end of 38 years of the Hospital for Natural Healing, there can be no doubt the founders, who kept the herbal educational torch burning for so long, would have been immensely pleased to know that in the twenty-first century, herbal practitioners graduate with science based BSc (Hons) degrees.

Albert Orbell retired from practice in 1975 and died peacefully in January 1986, age eighty-five years. His lifelong wish was that one of his family might follow in his footsteps, and he gained immense satisfaction and joy from seeing his grandson Kevin start formal herbal studies at the School of Herbal Medicine, Tunbridge Wells, in the autumn of 1985.

The story of Hydes Herbal Clinic, Leicester

Serene Foster

This chapter is based on an original interview with John Hyde in preparation for The Hydes Herbal Clinic Centenary in 2008 and further discussion with Arthur Hyde in 2014.

Hydes Herbal Clinic is the oldest and largest dedicated herbal clinic of its kind in England, surviving two world wars and the start of the NHS. It has been in continual operation since 1908, serving patients throughout Britain and abroad from its Leicester base. It serves as a platform for the professional delivery of the herbal consultation to the highest of clinical and ethical standards.

Its clinic ethos has always been that good herbal medicine must be backed up with good research and can only be delivered by rational clinical practice and a thorough approach. Hydes practitioners must be trained in the clinical practice of Western herbal medicine and have backgrounds in medicine and/or medical science research.

The story of Hydes is a fascinating one. Integral to the development of herbalism as a profession and, working at the core of the National Institute of Medical Herbalists (NIMH) for the majority of its existence, Hydes developed itself and in parallel fundamentally affected the shape and mission of NIMH as we know it today.

Hydes Herbal Clinic began with Jesse Hyde in a different age when 'folk medicine' was widely used. Universally available standardised medicine did not exist within the means of the majority of people, who had to take a greater role in their own healthcare.

Jesse Hyde originally ran a post office in Harrison Road, Leicester

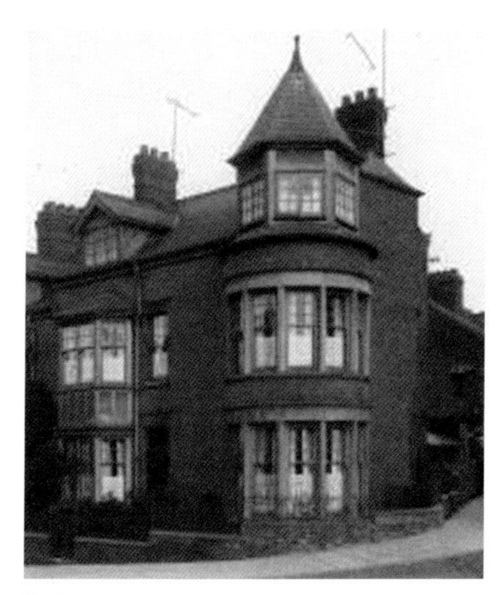

The first clinic in St Peter's Road Leicester

for 15 years and sold small packets of herbs in the late 1800s, to take as infusions. I find it quite heartwarming to picture a Victorian postmaster, upright and uniformed, acting as the point of primary healthcare for the community alongside all of his official duties. Jesse was committed to education and self-development, personal values which he sought to imbue in his children. He undertook training in medicine, botany and biology at night school. He firmly believed in a holistic approach to treatment focused on herbal imbibition but also, for example on 'physical manipulation' in which he was also a trained and respected practitioner. As a central figure in the community and a committed Christian, Mr Hyde was continually asked for help and as his reputation as an effective 'prescriber' became well known Jesse decided to break from his secure postal career and formed the area's first full-time Medical Herbal Clinic in St Peters Road in 1908, dedicated to health, to herbalism and 'doing things in the proper way' as he saw it.

Jesse determined that the proper approach should be medical, in that he would consult with patients to establish a medical history, perform a medical examination prior to diagnosis and prescription of herbs according to that patient's precise needs. Subsequent examination monitored the patient to ensure the appropriateness and efficacy of treatments, which could be adjusted as required. His scientific approach built from case histories a fuller understanding of the use of herbs in medical conditions. Key, as Jesse saw it, was that herbal preparations should be pure and of consistent strength. Whilst Jesse consulted in the front parlour, Maud, his wife, prepared herbal medicines in the annex. Husband and wife worked together in a truly family business.

With success the family business expanded. In 1911 Frederick Fletcher Hyde was born. Like his father, he was avid to learn and committed to self development. A brilliant scholar, he would gain three separate BSc degrees in Zoology, Chemistry and Botany, at a time before Herbalism was a degree level course in its own right. These were taught through Leicester College as externals from London and Bristol Universities whilst he worked with his father in the family business.

Frederick Fletcher Hyde (Fred) also lectured at the University of Leicester and co-founded its Pharmacology Department in the early 1930s. He met his wife Florence Annie when they both studied Botany. Florence herself went on to gain a first class BSc (Hons) and helped Fred in his plant research.

Whilst in the Pharmacy department Fred researched plants, with a particular objective in mind, having hit upon the new idea of processing plants into a liquid tincture to extract all the active constituents as a precursor to determining both the most appropriate 'imbibition' technique, and the most effective dosage quantity. In his research Fred worked through methods of comminution, imbibitions, maceration, concentration, maturity and filtration and came broadly to define the equivalent volume of raw herb required to produce one teaspoonful (5 ml) of processed tincture. Key to his innovation was that using measured quantities he could now control quality and strength at the point of production, thereby providing a more easily stored tincture to standardised potency. Hyde's production techniques led to more accurately dispensed and repeatable dosages.

This particular legacy is one of the many benefits which Hydes Herbal Clinic has contributed to the herbal industry, as the tincture method is today the predominant way Western herbal medicine patients take their herbal medicines. However, Hydes was also instrumental in forming much of the modern herbal practitioner's approach employed today. They were diligent record takers using measured performance indicators such as expressed lung capacity or the density of rash patterns to show progress, and as they standardised preparations for multiple patients they observed efficacy and adjusted formulae to tweak performance. Today we still retain examples of hand drawn charts and tables of readings from two generations ago.

Solid clinical experience of remedies and observation of real patients, whom Fred and his father treated over many years, confirmed their belief in herbal medicine as an invaluable and effective part of medicine in its totality. They also feared that a medical risk existed in allowing extracts from the whole active plant to be synthesised and replaced singularly by artificially produced chemicals, which could result in a situation where necessary components of the healing process are not

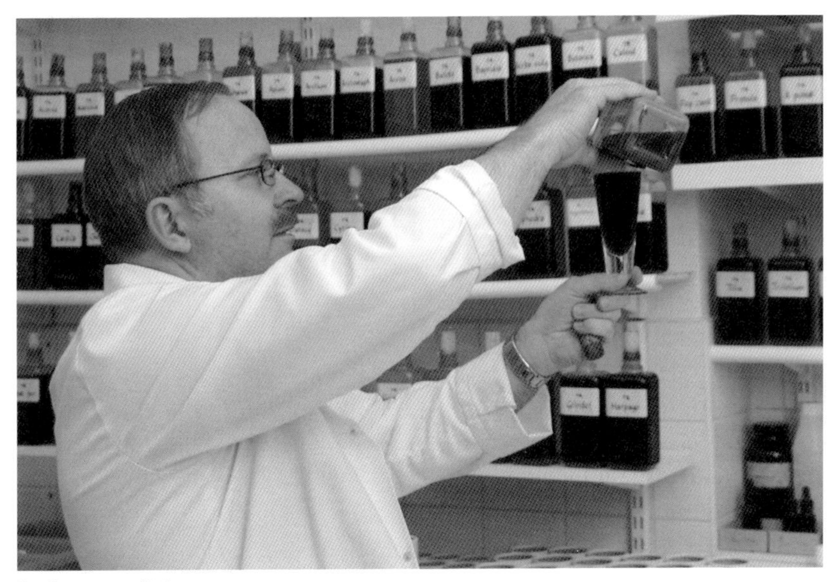

The dispensary at Hydes

absorbed properly by the body. They firmly believed that herbal medicine was 'nature's cocktail not the isolation of one active principle' and that the plant extracts were effective, natural and safe. Against the hedonism and confidence of the emerging pharmaceuticals industry, Hydes was a small brave voice but its message wasn't lost and is becoming ever more relevant as plant medicine is resurgent today.

Fred trained in diagnosis and examination at London University and it remains a key feature of Hydes Herbal Clinic today that we are conventionally medical in our approach and herbalist in our prescription. His core of professional belief was medical science not metaphysics.

Fred was also a key player in civic life and brought his influence to bear into the political arena. Herbal medicine has faced many challenges over the years since the charter of Henry VIII. In 1941 Hydes and others in response to public outcry tempered the Pharmacy and Medicines Act. Fred was keenly aware from this experience that his chosen profession would need to be fought for and protected. With the birth of the NHS in 1948 and 'free medicine for all' Hydes feared the end, but although herbalists weren't admitted to the mainstream, patients voted with their feet and within six months the consulting room was even busier than ever.

The 1968 Medicines Act was eventually more enlightened than the initial 1941 Act, and was instrumental in allowing herbalists to practise as we do today, although this was only after much struggle. There had initially been a move to restrict practice of herbal medicine to registered medical doctors, which given the low penetration of herbal knowledge amongst their ranks could well have been a fatal blow. Parliamentary discussion unanimously moved to accept the Act without division. However, Hydes and others mobilised and MPs received so many letters from patients that the Commons relented under an avalanche of post. Subsection 56 of the Act was therefore established to specify exemption for those properly qualified and practising as herbal practitioners. Fletcher was instrumental in working on that Act and serving on the Committees, discussing the detail of prescription and regulation, and championing the cause of herbal medicine. Frederick Fletcher Hyde was exceptional in his efforts in committee, and the example that he set by working hard in both mainstream medicine and herbal medicine. Fred's achievement was recognised in 2008 when the British Herbal Medicine Association presented Hydes an engraved plaque posthumously conferring its lifetime achievement award.

The practice grew so much in the 1930s that it moved to 68 London Road in 1934 where it still is today. Central of to the Hydes' life, this building combined clinic and family home for a number of years before becoming a dedicated clinic building some years later. Hydes remained fully operational during the Second World War, although Fred stepped up to additional civic duties and roles in the wartime Ministry of Works.

It was truly a family business as all the family collected herbs by hand from locations in rural Leicestershire including along the Grand Union Canal. Many family outings involved large hessian sacks used to bring vital raw material back to the Clinic. Father, as he was always known, would, as the diligent scientist, check all the herbs to ensure there were no errors in identification. Fletcher was a father committed to knowledge and his children would learn about the size and shape of the plants, and where they grow, identifying plants by leaf and stalk, collecting many herbs, from roots to tricky customers like nettles and thistles, and beyond that to the wildflowers such as daisy and dandelion. This form of harvest was safer back then as pesticide use was not excessive and streams and brooks cleaner for the gathering of aquatic herbs. The family also grew some of the rarer herbs in their garden and allotment, alongside their more conventional kitchen crops. It was an amazing sight which John Hyde remembered vividly.

> *"The top storey of the clinic used to be festooned with herbs, each leaf draped separately over string. It was a magical place, like a dried jungle, with fresh herb smells where you walked carefully in-between the trailing greenery. If it was a wet day or father was seeing patients, the herbs were processed. The naturally dried leaves were removed from stems and then chopped up into small pieces and processed into herbal medicine. In those days herbs were grown locally but now they are supplied from all over the world which means that we can ensure that we receive the very best quality and purity, insisting wherever possible that it is from an organic farm. That there is now an infrastructure of supply also means less danger of shortage outside of the peak season for natural harvest in the UK."*

The Hydes' household was crowded as clinic, tincture processing and domestic life meshed together in a common home. The large family room on the first floor was typical. Its dresser and shelves overcrowded with herbs and tinctures in jars, and medicines in various states of preparation jostling for space with ornaments, books, family photographs and the ephemera of daily living. This was the stimulating environment in which Fred's children lived and studied. Education, education, education was a 24/7 routine at Hydes a long time before modern politicians picked up the mantra.

John Hyde, born in 1943 studied Biochemistry, Botany, Materia Medica and Medicine spending some time as a medical student at Guy's Hospital in London, and several years at The London Hospital for Natural Healing and going on to achieve the highest marks ever given for the Entrance Examinations to the National Institute of Medical Herbalists. There was no formal degree in herbal medicine but it was clearly John's calling, if not his birthright. John chose the role of the clinician, dealing directly with patients and worked for over 40 years in the consulting room seeing thousands of patients. He also opened a consulting room in fashionable Mayfair only closing that when his own family responsibilities grew and his father began to slim down his practice with advancing age.

John is greatly responsible for Hydes Herbal Clinic as we see it today. Few practitioners will ever match his record of service to the community and he worked tirelessly to put herbalism into the public eye appearing on a number of TV programmes including *Midland's Today*, ATV's *The*

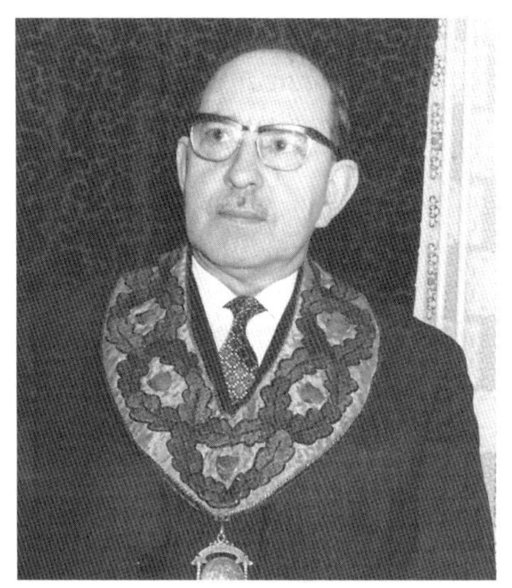

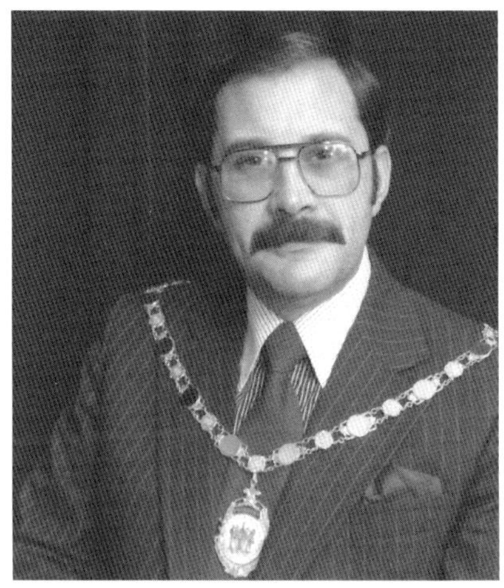

Frederick Fletcher Hyde (left) and John Hyde, both of whom were presidents of NIMH

Medicine Man, *Man Alive* for BBC2 and the series *Herbs for All* on Central TV.

John and his father, Fletcher, were also heavily involved in developing the National Institute of Medical Herbalists (NIMH) which since the 1860s has sought to further the cause of medical herbalism. This included key roles in developing young talent as the chairman of the board of examiners, furthering understanding as NIMH's press and public relations officer, and many years as a vice president. Both men served as president of the Institute. John Hyde's singular contribution as a dedicated medical herbalist was duly recognised in 1976 when was awarded a fellowship of the Institute for 'outstanding services to the profession', an honour which few have been privileged to hold.

John worked at Hydes together with his elder brother Arthur Hyde, who studied Agricultural Science at Cirencester, for 20 years until Arthur moved away and started a new practice. Arthur's original career aspirations were dramatically refocused by a serious motoring accident and by 1959 he was in Hydes full-time. He reapplied himself and passed the Institute's exams in a year, perhaps not surprisingly considering that all the young Hydes were 'brought up herbal'. Freya, their sister, choose not a practitioner role but worked in the back room with mother weighing herbs and preparing medicines whilst also pursuing her chosen vocation as a midwife. This would eventually take her, as a Senior Sister, out of the family clinic and away to Canada to a new life and family.

All the Hydes worked tirelessly to further medical herbalism committing valuable time to the NIMH Department of Education. Arthur and Fred lectured in Leicester and Sheffield. The Leicester Clinic took in aspiring practitioners for clinical practice and all the Hydes worked on NIMH fundraising. Quite a few of our senior colleagues will remember their experience at Hydes and some will even remember being a patient there. John Hyde once innovatively put on a benefit concert at the Albert Hall. Four generations of Hydes worked at the practice when John's son Mark worked in the Clinic for 15 years, and indeed John's daughter Rachel continues to work on the administrative side today.

Today's principal consultant is myself, Serene Foster who, with 30 years experience as a Medical Immunologist and as a Senior Research Scientist, worked under the direction of John Hyde for the first five years of my herbal career, ensuring that the chain of Hydes' influence was not broken. Although the last 'consulting Hyde' retired to an advisory capacity in 2003, there is a low staff turnover and the clinic still feels like a family firm. Indeed Serene's family now back up the full time staff when needed and everyone 'goes the extra mile' when required to do so, as a family would when it pulls together.

The Hydes Herbal Clinic story is a long one but it's as alive and fresh today as ever. Hydes Herbal Clinic congratulates NIMH on 150 years of service to the health of the public. Hydes commits itself to supporting NIMH in another 150 years of our vital mission to further the practice and extend the reach of the herbal medical profession.

Herbal Research

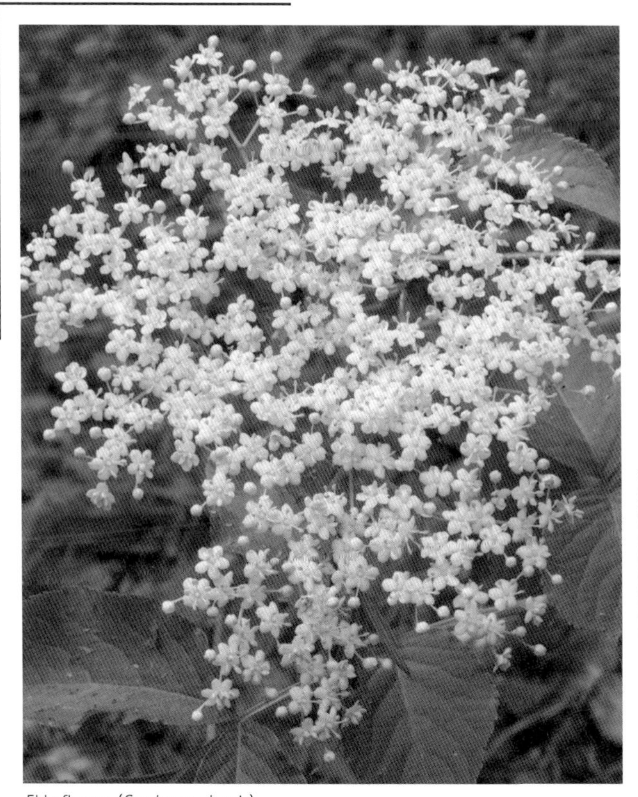

Elderflowers (*Sambucus nigra* L.)

The outlook for herbal medicine

Barbara Griggs

When I first embarked on a study of herbal medicine, some 40 years ago, I knew nothing whatever about my subject: at least, I had absolutely no practical experience of it, unless you count using a dock leaf to ease the smart of a nettle-sting. I grew up in the Cotswolds, in some of England's most beautiful countryside. Its herbal riches were part of my childhood scenery – hedgerows blooming with hawthorn and dog-roses and elderflowers, road-verges thick with yarrow and dandelion and cleavers, green meadows painted with cowslips and poppies; and underfoot, everywhere, the humble plantain. But when anyone in the family fell ill, no wise old grandmother brewed up herbal teas or salves to cure us: we called in Dr Duncan like everyone else.

Unlike France and most of our Continental neighbours, England lost touch with its traditions of herbal doctoring many years ago, for the most part brutally eradicated by the Industrial Revolution. Pockets of local knowledge survived, as Gabrielle Hatfield has painstakingly documented in her books, but by the 1960s, with new 'miracle' drugs flooding onto the market, dispensed free by our wonderful National Health Service, who needed that old grandmother stuff?

This was a view shared by practically everyone I knew, even in the hippie early 1970s. So lightheartedly embarking on a history of herbal medicine, along the lines of 'whatever happened to ...' I was surprised to find that there still seemed to be quite a lot of it about, a kind of green underground movement.

Doctors on the whole were ignorant of this older medicine. When in the late 1970s my husband was recovering in hospital from major surgery, I took him a bottle of that lovely Swiss herbal tonic, Biostrath.

Doctor after doctor, surprised not to see the mandatory Lucozade, commented sceptically on this herbal alternative. I asked one of them if he wasn't curious to know more about herbs. "If there were any useful medicines in herbs", he replied, "I reckon that we doctors would know about them and be using them."

My own friends were startled – even dismayed – by my choice of a subject for my next book. "Do you actually believe in herbs?" was a common query.

But by the 1990s, herbal medicine was forcing itself on the attention of doctors – and of the big pharmaceutical companies. Not only was there a very fast-growing market in over-the-counter herbal medicines – US sales alone were hitting the $2 billion mark by the mid-1990s – but clinical trials in Germany were giving a number of herbs the evidence-base that critics had always accused them of lacking. By the early 1990s, sales of herbal medicines in Germany alone already matched the whole US market, and preparations of ginkgo for the early stages of dementia, hypericum for mild depression, hawthorn and garlic for the heart were regularly being prescribed by German doctors.

The pharmaceutical companies woke up to find that far from the forgotten grandmother medicine they had once dismissed, herbs were now presenting formidable competition for some of their most important drugs. By 2001, two studies – admittedly small – had compared St John's wort with the two leading SSRI drugs, Prozac and Zoloft. In each, not only had the herb outperformed the pharmaceutical, but it had produced markedly fewer side-effects.

Alarmed, the medical establishment moved into the attack. Soon it was open season on herbal medicine. For the next decade and more, the pages of respected publications such as the *Journal of the American Medical Association* and the *New England Journal of Medicine*, as well as popular newspapers and magazines, featured what increasingly came to seem like a well-organised campaign to discredit herbal medicine – particularly those which represented a real threat to the sales of blockbuster drugs.

In 1998, the cover of Time magazine showed a colourful montage of ginkgo, St John's wort, echinacea and ginseng, with the line: 'It's great business but is it good for what ails us?' (*Time* 1998). The story inside featured the grave misgivings of responsible physicians about the safety, efficacy and potential misuse of herbal products. In 2001 JAMA ran a study (sponsored by the makers of Zoloft) showing that for people suffering from major depression – for which nobody had ever suggested that St John's wort might be effective – the herb performed no better than placebo: the study produced headlines all over the US press claiming that St John's wort was useless for depression (Shelton *et al.* 2001). Other stories suggested that taking it could give you cataracts. 'Echinacea may be dangerous for children, warns watchdog' and 'Herb cures that "do you more harm than good"' were typical newspaper headlines.

The internet hosted numbers of Quackbuster sites, featuring shrill denunciations of CAM. In 2004 The Skeptic (http://www.skeptic.org.uk/) warned 'Herbal medicine is a pseudoscientific approach to healthcare and healing. It is based on mystical thinking and there is little quality scientific evidence to support the claims of its efficacy'.

Professor R. Barker Bausell, one-time Research Director for the Complementary and Alternative Medicine Research Center of the US National Institutes of Health, put it categorically in his 2007 book *Snake Oil Science*: 'There is no compelling credible scientific evidence to suggest that any CAM therapy benefits any medical condition or reduces any medical symptom (pain or otherwise) better than a placebo' (Barker Bausell 2007).

Herbs, in other words, don't work.

One of the most outrageous examples of this approach was published in the UK *Journal of Postgraduate Medicine*, entitled *A systematic review of randomised clinical trials of individualised herbal medicine in any indication* (Guo *et al.* 2007). The authors – they included Professor Edzard Ernst, longtime outspoken critic of all forms of CAM – found precisely three studies worthy of their attention: the longest ran for no more than 6 months, the other two merely a few weeks. On the basis of this, the authors solemnly dismissed centuries of traditional medical practice from around the world, concluding that '...there is no convincing evidence supporting its use in any indication'.

Another charge against herbal medicine constantly aired in the media was that that because herbs had never been properly tested, they were potentially extremely dangerous. It was always hard to flesh out this accusation with actual statistics: but there were certainly abundant statistics demonstrating just how harmful pharmaceutical drugs could be, especially in a hospital setting. The figures – receiving more and more media attention as the new century advanced – were and are horrendous.

Adverse reactions to prescribed drugs send hundreds of thousands of people to hospital every year, killing significant numbers of them, and the toll is rising annually. According to a 2004 study, at any time the equivalent of up to seven 800-bed hospitals in the UK was likely to be occupied by patients suffering from an adverse drug reaction (Pirmohamed *et al.* 2004). A single drug can produce a shocking death toll: in November 2004 the US Food and Drug Administration estimated that Merck's arthritis blockbuster drug Vioxx had probably contributed to over 27,000 heart attacks and sudden cardiac deaths between 1993 and 2003. In the US today, fatal reactions to prescribed drugs caused 106,000 deaths (US DHSS 2012).

Critics of herbal medicine have always emphasised how little scientific evidence there was that it worked – unlike pharmaceutical drugs which met the 'gold standard' of proper clinical trials, to constitute evidence-based medicine. But the much-vaunted evidence base of pharmaceuticals has been crumbling over the last few years: its deficiencies exposed not by indignant herbalists but by doctors, research scientists and journalists studying the hard evidence. One-time editor of *The New England Journal of Medicine*, Marcia Angell published a hard-hitting expose of the growing corruption in the pharmaceutical industry in 2004, called 'The Truth About The Drug Companies'. More recently, she has commented that 'It is simply no longer possible to believe much of the clinical research that is published, or to rely on the judgment of trusted physicians or authoritative medical guidelines. I take no pleasure in this conclusion, which I reached slowly and reluctantly over my two decades as an editor' (Angell 2009).

For years now antidepressants have been among the biggest earners for the pharmaceutical industry. In 2008, a clinical psychologist, Professor Irving Kirsch and fellow researchers used the Freedom of Information Act to obtain the data on all clinical trials submitted to the FDA for the licensing of four new-generation anti-depressants. The meta-analysis they published in the *PLOS Medicine Journal* of February 26 that year showed that people got better on medication – but they also got better on placebo, and the difference between the two was so small that it fell below the criterion for clinical significance established by NICE (Kirsch *et al.* 2008).

Tamiflu, which the NHS has spent over £500,000 stockpiling against a catastrophic flu epidemic, was not much better than money down the drain. An analysis by the Cochrane Collaboration showed that the drug does not, in fact, reduce the number of hospitalisations; that there is no real evidence of a benefit when pneumonia develops; and that at the most it might take a few hours off the duration of flu symptoms – all this at a cost of some fairly unpleasant side-effects in a few of those taking it.

Among the loudest critics of 'unscientific' medicine is journalist Dr Ben Goldacre, whose columns in the *Guardian* regularly took a swipe at herbal medicine, among other favourite targets such as homeopathy and nutritional supplements. Most recently he has published a damning attack on the pharmaceutical industry, called *Bad pharma: how drug companies mislead doctors and harm patients* (Goldacre 2012).

Publications like these, generating the same kind of headlines and media attention as herbal horror stories once did, have been eating away at public confidence in wonder drugs for some time now, although the *Daily Express* (2014) still loyally comes up with excitable front-page headlines: *NEW WAY TO END ARTHRITIS PAIN: Simple jab has no side effects.*

Decades of adverse publicity, however, appear to have had little impact on public attitudes to herbal medicine. An Ipsos Mori poll commissioned by the MHRA in 2009 showed an astonishingly high level of public support. More than a quarter of the population had bought over-the-counter herbal medicines in the previous two years: 1 in 20 had consulted a practitioner of Traditional Chinese Medicine; 1 in 12 had consulted a practitioner of Western herbal medicine.

Friends, I notice, no longer ask me whether I 'believe' in herbal medicine. (A herbalist friend of mine, when asked this question, retorts 'Do you believe in food?'). Instead they ring up to ask whether I can suggest anything for their migraine, for their asthma, for their intractable insomnia, for a teenage son's devastating acne, for a favourite aunt's crippling arthritis. When I suggest a visit to a medical herbalist, I am often asked to suggest one – and later find that they actually went.

Over the centuries, herbal medicine has flourished when mainstream medicine seemed either out of reach to all but the wealthy – as in Elizabethan times – or else dangerously ineffectual – as in the early nineteenth century, when purging, bleeding and mercury constituted its main therapies. The crisis facing Western medicine today is partly a financial one. Because of the huge and growing burden of caring for the chronically ill, national health budgets are being strained to breaking point. The outlook for Britain's National Health Service is bleak indeed as it struggles to face a funding shortfall running into billions of pounds. In February 2014, Sir David Nicholson, on the eve of his retirement as Chief Executive of NHS England, warned that unless drastic measures were taken, the NHS could face a shortfall of £30 billion by 2021 (*Daily Telegraph* 2014).

But the problems confronting the NHS – and Western medicine generally – are not just financial, crippling though these are likely to become. The much more serious problem is this: the reductionist one-disease one-drug approach is simply not very good at treating complex chronic disease. Chronic diseases of every kind are everywhere and on the rise: the global economic impact of the five leading non-communicable diseases – cardiovascular disease, chronic respiratory disease, cancer, diabetes and mental ill-health – could total US$ 47 trillion over the next 20 years, according to a study released in 2011 by the World Economic Forum (Bloom *et al* 2011).

Over decades of advance, Western medicine has come up with an arsenal of useful drugs, for many of which herbal medicines can be no substitute. But arthritis, asthma, metabolic syndrome, inflammatory bowel disease and all such chronic conditions are not tidy straightforward disorders which a powerful single-molecule single drug can sort out. Anxiety, digestive problems, sleep disorders, high cholesterol, high blood pressure may all present alongside the main problem in a single patient, who is likely to end up swallowing 10 or 12 different pills – and trying to cope with the accumulating side effects.

Any of these problems are likely to involve multiple tissues and organ systems, and as US herbalist and Kevin Spelman (2007) puts it, 'a system-wide disorder will need a system-wide therapy ... The human genome has been selected to respond to low-dose, complex mixtures of plant compounds. Seven to ten million years of human evolutionary history should make it obvious that exposure to one chemical at a time has no precedent in human history ...'

Herbal medicines are precisely that: low-dose complex mixtures of dozens of different phytochemicals, which can interact simultaneously with multiple compounds or processes in the human body. Garlic, for instance, has antibiotic, antiparasitic, antiviral and antifungal, expectorant, non-sedating antihistamine, anticoagulant, hypotensive, antithrombic and vasodilator activity – and I could go on. Complex diseases, in other words, will respond best to complex medicines.

James Duke, one of America's leading experts on botanical medicine, puts it beautifully: 'Unlike synthetic pharmaceuticals, herbs and spices each offer the sick human body a menu of thousands of biologically active evolutionarily familiar phytochemicals from which I believe the body extracts those it needs to bring it back into balance...' (Duke 2010).

As biochemical research gives us more and more insights into the extraordinary complexity of the human body, and the multiple ways in which it interacts with the thousands of phytochemicals that the plant world offers us, it is becoming clear that herbal medicine has science on its side. This is future medicine.

The question people may be asking each other tomorrow will perhaps be: "Do you believe in drugs?"

References

Angell, M., 2009. Drug companies and doctors: a story of corruption. [online]. New York review of books. Available from: http://www.nybooks.com/articles/archives/2009/jan/15/drug-companies-doctorsa-story-of-corruption/ [Accessed 19 July 2014].

Barker Bausell, R., 2007. *Snake Oil Science*. Oxford University Press. p. 254.

Bloom, D.E., *et al.* 2011. The global economic burden of non-communicable diseases. Geneva. World Economic Forum.

Goldacre, B., 2012. *Bad Pharma*. London: Fourth Estate.

Greenwald, J., 1998. ***Herbal healing*** [online], Time. Available from: http://content.time.com/time/world/article/0,8599,2054090,00.html [Accessed 19 July 2014].

Guo, R., Canter, P.H. and Ernst, E. 2007. A systematic review of randomised clinical trials of individiualized herbal medicine in any indication. *Postgraduate medical journal*. 83, 633–7.

Kirsch, I., *et al.*, 2008. Initial severity and antidepressant benefits: a meta-analysis of data submitted to the Food and Drug Administration. *PLOS medicine*. February. 5(2), e45, 0260–7.

Nicholson, D., 2014. 'NHS to adapt to survive', says chief executive. ***Daily Telegraph***, 11 February, 2014.

Pirmohamed, M., *et al.*, 2004. Adverse drug reactions as cause of admission to hospital: prospective analysis of 18,820 patients. *British medical journal*. 329(15).

Reynolds, M., 2014. New drugs could stop misery of arthritis for 8 million Britons *Daily Express*, 18 June, 2014.

Shelton, R.C., *et al.*, 2001. Effectiveness of St John's wort in major depression: a randomized controlled trial. *Journal of the American Medical Association*. 18 April. 285(15),1978–86.

Spelman, K., 2007. Preventative measures for metabolic syndrome. *Unified health*. 3, 30–8.

US DHSS., 2012. National vital statistics report. 61, 1–52.

Further reading

Griggs, B. 1981. Green pharmacy: a history of Western herbal medicine. London: Jill Norman & Hobhouse.

Griggs, B. 1997. *New green pharmacy: the story of Western herbal medicine.* London: Vermilion.

Griggs, B. 1986. *The food factor: why we are what we eat.* London: Viking.

Griggs, B. 1993. *The green witch: a modern woman's herbal.* London: Vermillion.

Griggs, B. 2008. *Helpful herbs for health and beauty.* Oxford: Infinite Ideas.

Herbal practice: just how complex an intervention?

Alison Denham

Abstract

What do herbalists do? The public often have little idea, but do we? There has been little published research into just what herbal practice is, and here I would like to give some pointers towards the design of research studies which might help to share knowledge within the profession. These suggestions are based on my experience as part of the team which carried out a pilot randomised waiting-list controlled study of the care by herbalists of women in the menopausal transition. The clinical encounter is complex, many-faceted, and defies description, but in the design of research studies it is necessary to explore how there can be some consistency between practitioners. We need to find more ways of sharing our clinical expertise and experience in a structured way so that, if a given treatment is shown to be successful or unsuccessful, the reader can understand what treatment was given. The concept of the complex intervention which attempts to encompass the numerous aspects of any clinical encounter, is used here to discuss research studies into traditional acupuncture which could help in planning studies in herbal practice. Finally, I propose that qualitative studies could help in this process.

Introduction

After 30 years in clinical practice, it is still frustrating to me that so many people have no idea what medical herbalists do. Within our profession, we know that we take a clinical history which is extremely broad and variable, we may examine the patient, we discuss an array of factors such as diet, lifestyle, exercise, food supplements, emotional and spiritual meaning even as we are formulating a diagnostic rationale for our treatment plan and eventually, after all that, compose the individualised prescription (Conway 2011). There is therefore substantial diversity between consultations, between practitioners and between prescriptions. This is all as it should be, but is problematic when we come to try to share our experience within the profession, to evaluate our practice or to explain our practice to the wider world. Consultations form a private space which is determined by and determines our personal experience, but to learn we must also share knowledge.

Reflecting on a choice of topic for this chapter took me back to the most challenging activity into which NIMH drew me: 'Changing with Herbs', a pilot, randomised waiting-list controlled study of the care of women in the menopausal transition. The team included the lead researcher Julia Green, Sue Hawkey, myself and the statisticians at the Research and Development Support Unit of the United Bristol Healthcare Trust. One day when Julia rang about a problem, I had a vision as from the Hitchcock thriller *North by Northwest* of me holding onto the edge of a cliff by my fingertips with Julia holding on to me – we felt so far from any secure place as we were not part of an established research team. However, with the input of the statisticians we achieved our objective, and published our study in a recognised peer-reviewed journal. Using the validated Greene Climacteric Scale, we found a statistically and clinically significant reduction in menopausal symptoms in the treatment group (15 women) compared to the control group (30 women) over a six-month period (Green *et al.* 2007). The control group were then offered treatment and a total of 35 women (aged 46–58) were treated, and our later paper discussed the prescriptions composed by the three NIMH herbalists involved in the study (Denham *et al.* 2011).

We chose to investigate the whole care given by herbalists, in conventional parlance the 'complex intervention', and our experience could help researchers in the planning of future qualitative studies or clinical trials. To evaluate the whole 'package of care' is a valid goal, in that feedback from the patients in our study was that they valued the communication engendered within the consultation. A recent study of 19 patients who consulted herbalists found that they considered that the collaboration between patient and practitioner was a crucial element underpinning the success of herbal medicine (Little 2009). The results of this qualitative study suggest it was the variability and individuality of the consultations and treatments that patients regarded as important. However, the external validity (the extent to which the results of our clinical trial might hold for patients who consulted other herbalists), and reproducibility (repeatability) of the results of any pilot study or clinical trial depend on whether the whole treatment, the so-called complex intervention, can be reproduced (MacPherson *et al.* 2013a). If there were to be a future clinical trial, there would have to be further discussion of this alarmingly complex 'complex intervention'.

Issues in trial design in herbal practice

Research is not about justifying ourselves as a profession, showing that herbs 'work,' it is about sharing clinical experience and this chapter focusses on the care given by practitioners involved in clinical trials. To evaluate the results of any published research, the practitioner needs to know what treatment was given.

There are many other issues in trial design in any clinical practice, such as the recruitment of participants, the influence of the setting, the length of the trial, the way in which results are measured, and the funding. Given the limited funding and resources available, methodological questions are central to making best use of the resources available and thus developing a research culture in complementary medicine. It is important that the quality of any research justifies the input of patients, practitioners and funders. For example, sometimes in trials of herbal medicinal products, there are too few participants for the results to be statistically significant.

Complex interventions

This debate over the characterisation of complex interventions is not unique to herbal practice and, since we began planning our pilot study in 1998, there has been an ever expanding literature on the evaluation of clinical practice in complementary medicine (Boon *et al.* 2007). This debate on the evaluation of complex interventions in healthcare builds on the Medical Research Council (MRC) guidance originally published in 2000 and updated in 2008 (Craig *et al.* 2013, MRC 2008). This has led to increased understanding of the nature of complex interventions, and the different ways in which the components of any care can be conceptualised (Clark 2013, Cohn *et al.* 2013, Datta and Petticrew 2013).

Much of this research is in the area of health promotion (for example, programmes of care for people who have had a heart attack), mental health (such as programmes of psychotherapy or to promote qualities such as self-esteem) and social care (programmes to support children's early learning). However, although the context would be different, this does mean that it would now be possible to design a clinical trial of herbal practice building on both the experience and theoretical work of these researchers. Reading the reports of these clinical trials would help any future researcher to think carefully about the detailed aspects of the design of the proposed clinical trial.

The consultation

Although there has been little research into the clinical practice of herbalists, there has been relevant research in traditional acupuncture. Paterson and Dieppe (2005) confronted the question of whether elements of the treatment could be investigated separately from the consultation process. They argued that when the consultation is a process which gradually engenders the diagnosis, in the sense of the rationale for treatment, then the elements of the process cannot be separated. A recent randomised, controlled trial in which 755 patients were treated for depression by acupuncture, counselling or usual care, has led to three relevant papers which analyse the treatments given by the 23 acupuncturists in the trial, and the way in which a protocol was designed for the treatments given in the trial (MacPherson *et al.* 2013b). A consensus process was used to identify the components of acupuncture in the treatment of depression in order to define the scope of the proposed complex intervention in the forthcoming clinical trial. The 15 acupuncturists who took part in the consensus process represented a range of theoretical and educational backgrounds, and were able to agree on 16 elements of the consultation/treatment and on a list of theoretical frameworks, lifestyle advice and additional techniques (MacPherson and Schroer 2007). A pilot study on 40 patients incorporated a range of methods including interviews with patients, acupuncturists and medical practitioners to understand the proposed study in depth and to ensure that the trial procedures felt credible to the acupuncturists (Schroer *et al.* 2012). After further consultation with the acupuncturists who would be treating patients in the trial, the research team finalised a manual which listed the treatment processes and a practitioner logbook. In the trial, 23 acupuncturists delivered 2,741 treatment sessions for the 266 patients in the treatment group and the process was a success in that 22 of the acupuncturists felt able to provide care either exactly the same as or similar to their normal care (Macpherson *et al.* 2013a). The relevance to herbal practice is that acupuncture is also a profession which encompasses different treatment approaches, and includes a detailed consultation and discussion of care with the patient. While the detail would be different, it would be possible to use the same methods to seek some consensus amongst herbal practitioners when planning a clinical trial.

The prescription

If some consensus is sought on the treatments given by the practitioners taking part in a pragmatic randomised controlled trial, there is a balance to be found between retaining the variability of everyday clinical practice and defining the clinical single intervention. One could design a standard formula but this would not reflect normal practice. A survey of 378 herbal practitioners in Australia found that 97 per cent dispensed their own prescriptions, and 87 per cent prepared individualised herbal prescriptions (Casey *et al.* 2007). In our study, the practitioners prescribed freely, and a total of 80 herbs were used to treat the 35 participants with menopausal symptoms. The three practitioners had trained together and a larger number of practitioners, treating a larger population, would certainly use more herbs. When exploring the herbs used, I was struck that some herbs which I use regularly were not mentioned.

However, there were some frontrunners (which I do use!) including *Leonurus cardiaca* L. and *Salvia officinalis* L. – which suggests that a list of herbs could be developed through consensus amongst the practitioners involved in a future clinical trial. In particular in our study, there was variation between the herbalists in the number of additional prescriptions for sleeping, coughs and colds and so on. There could have been more consistency between practitioners without unduly compromising patient care. Again, there has been relevant research in the field of traditional acupuncture. Macpherson *et al.* (2006) described the clinical practice of six acupuncturists who treated 148 patients in a randomised controlled trial of traditional acupuncture for low back pain. They found it was possible to achieve some concordance on the diagnostic categories, but also showed that 177 different acupuncture points were used.

Diet and nutritional advice

Discussion of lifestyle is integral to herbal medicine as the aim of the consultation is to enable the patient to take responsibility for changes in health. A survey of 378 herbalists in Australia found that over 80 per cent gave nutritional advice as part of the consultation (Casey *et al.* 2008), and the results of our study were similar. Each woman was given a diet sheet at the first consultation, and specific aspects of diet were discussed in 25 per cent of the consultations. One could argue that the volume and range of discussion on diet, nutrition and food supplements was a major confounding factor in the interpretation of the results of our study. However, the extent to which each participant followed the advice is unknown, which means that the characterisation and thus reproducibility of the intervention is unclear.

Again looking at acupuncture, a study of the discussion and advice given by six traditional acupuncturists in a randomised controlled trial of the treatment of chronic low back pain found that advice was an integral part of the intervention as it was chosen with regard to the diagnosis and theoretical underpinning of the intervention for the individual patient (MacPherson and Thomas 2008). The same argument can be made in herbal practice in that change in diet is one of the ways in which herbal practitioners aim to improve the vitality of the patient. It is inseparable from normal clinical practice and giving standard advice would not be normal care in herbal practice. Having said this, it would indeed be helpful for the practitioners in a future clinical trial to reach a greater consensus on the discussion of diet and food supplements. However, this caution would be applicable in many clinical settings in that the consumption of food supplements is widespread and could be an unknown factor in many clinical trials. In the case of menopausal symptoms, foods and food supplements which contain phytoestrogens may or may not have an effect (Bolanos *et al.* 2010), but they are widely consumed (Daley *et al.* 2006). This could be a confounding factor in any future clinical trial as it could be difficult to recruit a population of menopausal women who had not already experimented with food supplements or changes in diet.

What can we learn about trial design in herbal practice?

We learned some important points – first that it was possible to recruit in a primary care setting, and thus evaluate holistic herbal practice in that context. Second, we aimed to make our study replicable and used a validated outcome measure, the Greene Climacteric Scale, which is widely used throughout the world (Greene 2008; Vasconcelos-Raposo *et al.* 2012). This questionnaire proved to be sensitive to change in severity of symptoms, and thus it means that our study adds to the literature as it can be directly compared with other clinical studies. A weakness of our study, in some eyes, was that it was a waiting-list study. The control group was made of women who waited 16 weeks before being offered the same course of treatment. This method has been increasingly used in areas where it is impossible to make a 'dummy' treatment, for example, cognitive behaviour therapy (Cuijpers *et al.* 2014). It is too large a topic to go into here, but it must be remembered that many researchers consider that use of a waiting-list or non-treatment group introduces a bias as treatment confers a benefit just by being treatment (Fregni *et al.* 2010). This issue further heightens the importance of ensuring that other aspects of trial design are carefully considered.

Qualitative studies

A first step in designing any future study would be to model the intervention using qualitative methods (Datta and Petticrew 2013). This could build on the experience of researchers in traditional acupuncture. It would, for example, be possible for a group of herbalists to agree parameters on the length and structure of the consultation. The acupuncturists involved in the study on depression discussed above kept a logbook, and another means of understanding the clinical reasoning process during the consultation would be for practitioners to keep narrative dairies. This process was used in the context of a community based strategy to improve maternal care after childbirth and reduce postnatal depression (Hawe *et al.* 2004), and would be helpful in uncovering differences in consultation style and content. This would strengthen the profession, rather than lead to conformity, as it would help us to explore the significance of the consultation.

Qualitative study of the consultation style of practitioners could make it possible to identify themes in herbal practice. As part of her ethnographic study of the practice of herbal medicine, Nina Nissen (2011) investigated the way in which herbalists perceived the meaning of holism, and suggested that the way in which this central concept was described could be visualised according to three perspectives: homeostatic, bio-psycho-social and spiritual. Each perspective may be associated with variations in practice, yet maybe there is a common quality of herbal practice: that the herbs are just part of the relationship constructed between patient and practitioner. T to quote one of the herbalists interviewed: 'simply encouraging someone to go dancing again. And that could be the way in which that person releases or finds fulfilment or finds wholeness, actually...' (Nissen and Evans 2012, p. 10). Equally, the herbs have their own meaning which is highlighted in a brief report of an ongoing ethnographic study of the profession by Guy Waddell (2013). I am supervising an MSc student at UCLan who is undertaking a study which asks practitioners to record their thinking while preparing prescriptions. Another student is planning a dissertation in which the rationale for prescribing will be discussed by herbalists. These studies will add to the small evidence base surrounding current herbal practice in Britain, and help practitioners to understand more about practice. Although this brings us into the world of conflicting models of healthcare research – daunting but exciting – my motivation in research has been to share knowledge: to perceive ourselves as a profession, then we must share knowledge through publications. Yet, to be authentic in any sense, research must engage with the lived experience of practice.

References

Bolanos, R., Del, C. and Francia, J. 2010. Soy isoflavones versus placebo in the treatment of climacteric vasomotor symptoms: Systematic review and meta-analysis. *Menopause.* 17, 660–6.

Boon, H., *et al.*, 2007. Evaluating complex healthcare systems: A critique of four approaches. *Evidence based complementary and alternative medicine.* 4(3), 279–85.

Casey, M., Adams, J. and Sibbritt, D. 2007. An examination of the prescription and dispensing of medicines by Western herbal therapists: A national survey in Australia. *Complementary therapies in medicine.* 15(1), 3–20.

Casey, M., Adams, J. and Sibbritt, D. 2008. An examination of the clinical practices and perceptions of professional herbalists providing patient care concurrently with conventional medical practice in Australia. *Complementary therapies in medicine.* 16(4), 228–32.

Clark, A. 2013. What are the components of complex interventions in healthcare? Theorizing approaches to parts, powers and the whole intervention. *Social science in medicine.* 93, 185–93.

Cohn, S., *et al.* 2013. Entangled complexity: why complex interventions are just not complicated enough. *Journal of health service research and policy.* 18(1), 40–3.

Conway, P. 2011. *The consultation in phytotherapy.* Edinburgh: Churchill Livingstone.

Craig, P. *et al.*, 2013. Developing and evaluating complex interventions: the new Medical Research Council guidance. *International journal of nursing studies.* 50(5), 587–92.

Cuijpers, P., *et al.*, 2014. Psychological treatment of generalized anxiety disorder: A meta-analysis. *Clinical psychology review.* 34(2), 130–40.

Daley, A., *et al.*, 2006. Factors associated with the use of complementary medicine and non-pharmacological interventions in symptomatic menopausal women. *Climacteric.* 9(5), 336–46.

Datta, J. and Petticrew, M. 2013. Challenges to evaluating complex interventions: A content analysis of published paper. *BMC public health.* 13, 568.

Denham, A., Green, J. and Hawkey, S. 2011. What's in the bottle? Prescriptions formulated by medical herbalists in a clinical trial of treatment during the menopause. *Journal of herbal medicine.* 1(3–4), 95–101.

Fregni, F., *et al.*, 2010. Challenges and recommendations for placebo controls in randomized trials in physical and rehabilitation medicine: A report of the international placebo symposium working group. *American journal of physical and medical rehabilitation.* 89(2), 160–72.

Green, J., *et al.*, 2007. Treatment of menopausal symptoms by qualified herbal practitioners: A prospective, randomized controlled trial. *Family practice.* 24(5), 468–74.

Greene, J. 2008. Constructing a standard climacteric scale. *Maturitas.* 61(1–2), 78–84.

Hawe, P., Shiell, A., Riley, T. and Gold, L. (2004) Methods for exploring implementation variation and local context within a cluster randomised community intervention trial. *Journal of epidemiology and community health.* 58(9), 788–93.

Little, C. 2009. Simply because it works better: exploring motives for the use of medical herbalism in contemporary UK health care. *Complementary therapies in medicine.* 17(5–6), 300–8.

MacPherson, H., Thorpe, L. and Thomas, K. 2006. Beyond needling – therapeutic processes in acupuncture care: a qualitative study nested within a low-back pain trial. *Journal of alternative and complementary medicine.* 12(9), 873–80.

MacPherson, H. and Schroer, S. 2007. Acupuncture as a complex intervention for depression: a consensus method to develop a standardised treatment protocol for a randomised controlled trial. *Complementary therapies in medicine.* 15(2), 92–100.

MacPherson, H. and Thomas, K. 2008. Self-help advice as a process integral to traditional acupuncture care: implications for trial design. *Complementary therapies in medicine.* 16(2), 101–6.

MacPherson, H., *et al.*, 2013a. Acupuncture for depression: patterns of diagnosis and treatment within a randomised controlled trial. *Evidence based complementary and alternative medicine.* 2013, 286048.

MacPherson, H., *et al.*, 2013b. Acupuncture and counselling for depression in primary care: a randomised controlled trial. *PLoS Medicine.* 10(9), e1001518.

Medicines Research Council (2008) *Complex Interventions guidance* [online] accessed on 2 April 2014 at: http://www.mrc.ac.uk/Utilities/Documentrecord/index.htm?d=MRC004871.

Nissen, N. 2011. Perspectives on holism in the contemporary practice of Western herbal medicine in the UK. *Journal of herbal medicine.* 1(3–4), 76–82.

Nissen, N. and Evans, S. 2012. Exploring the practice and use of Western herbal medicine: perspectives from the social science literature. *Journal of herbal medicine.* 2(1), 6–15.

Paterson, C. and Dieppe, P. 2005. Characteristic and incidental (placebo) effects in complex interventions such as acupuncture. *British medical journal.* 330(7501), 1202–5.

Schroer, S., *et al.*, J. 2012. Acupuncture for depression: exploring model validity and the related issue of credibility in the context of designing a pragmatic trial. *CNS neuroscience and therapeutics.* 18(4), 318–26.

Vasconcelos-Raposo, J., *et al.*, C. 2012. Factor structure and normative data of the Greene Climacteric Scale among postmenopausal Portuguese women. *Maturitas.* 72(3), 256–62.

Waddell, G., *et al.*,. 2013. A multi-sited ethnography of the professional practice of Western herbal medicine by medical herbalists in the UK. *European journal of integrative medicine.* 5(6), 577–8.

More than the sum of their parts
An art and a science – how little we know

Paul Chenery

Introduction

The recent history of medicine has been about the elucidation of the molecular mechanisms of disease, in order to seek molecular answers in pharmaceutics. Yet, the physiological action of species one upon another (including the action of plant species on humans and animals, in other words 'herbal activity') is as old as life itself and is one of the fundamental realities of evolutionary biology. The latest thrust of drug companies is to develop medicines tailor-made for individuals based on their genomes, something that has always been basic to herbal medicine, albeit from a non-molecular viewpoint. So modern human understanding may be converging, often from opposite poles, in order to develop a greater understanding of aspects of the same problem.

This article describes bio-molecular factors that were uncovered during the investigation of anthroposophical methods of determining vitality. Here is outlined how simple physiochemical principles of inter-facial phenomena and micro-emulsification, which are extremely well known in basic pharmaceutical drug design, not only underlie plant competitive strategy, but are also transmitted into herbalists' tinctures by co-surfactance. This suggests a reason why tinctures have proved so successful and enduringly popular with professional practitioners, despite the technical development of many other forms of, often more convenient, herbal extract. Our plants have evolved over millions of years to survive into the current era only due to their increasing levels of sophisticated competitive strategies. These involve the production of botanical molecules that affect physiological pathways in other species (well defined by drug researchers and which are sometimes called 'xenobiotics') but, equally importantly, plants have simultaneously harnessed the forces of molecular nature to physically 'deliver' these valuable compounds in the most efficient ways possible. These ways depend on the watery milieu and so are frequently modified by dehydration, but are also very often optimised by alcohol and water extraction.

Medicines may work at many levels simultaneously, from the cellular to the spiritual. Some would hold that modern herbal medicine, because it is predominantly physiological and yet also fundamentally connected to the natural world through its immediate derivation and origin, is overall the best placed system to help reconnect modern humanity to its lost roots. A broad philosophical basis for this has been proposed by HRH The Prince of Wales (2010), a keen champion of herbal medicine. It has also been suggested that increasing our knowledge of shared signals between plants and animals may be one way of aiding the understanding of herbal medicine (Schulz 2002).

Physiological actions of plants on people

Despite the enormous strides taken by science in unravelling the physiological interactions between plants and people, the very complexity of this defies complete elucidation. So we rely greatly on empirical data – the evidence that over generations our medicines have been found to work. Fortunately for those working to bring forward licenses for herbal medicinal products to compete with licensed synthetic drugs, the relevant Directive (Europe 2004) under which we in Europe currently live, accepts this world view and allows that adequate tradition is itself sufficient evidence for the safety and efficacy of traditional medicines.

Much of the science involved with unravelling herbal action has concentrated on molecular phenomena, how certain biochemical or phytochemical molecular groups can be seen to have an action upon systems that feed back into pathophysiological, or disease, states. A great deal of information on this now exists and several major works over the past 15 years or so have brought together and made accessible in one place for the first time, modern world-wide information on the bio-molecular bases of empirical physiological interaction between plants and people, principally at a cellular level (Mills and Bone 2000, Mills and Bone 2005, ESCOP 2010).

There is also scientific information from which it may be inferred that herbal medicine in general is extremely well designed through natural evolution to simultaneously optimise activity on several planes of activity. As explained below, there are clear and well understood evolutionary mechanisms at play. By studying the bases underlying such mechanisms better, herbalists may be able to improve the art and science of herbal medicine.

In order to better understand the bigger picture of how physiology operates on many different levels at once, it is possible to draw up diagrammatic matrices in which these activities occur in different horizontal and vertical axes of complex dynamic interactions. Lapraz *et al.* (2012) have pioneered the development of this line of reasoning into a complete system of medicine, an approach which they call 'endobiogenie'. In this model endocrine feedback is the biochemical 'railway' network ultimately linking all physiological stations.

Appropriate formulations and dosages: Getting round natural defence systems

One of the fundamental necessities of living systems is that they develop and maintain powerful defences. It is when these defence systems are overwhelmed or malfunction, that medicine is required. We do, however, also need to overcome defences to deliver medicines to the right place. The first line of defence is the skin. We are familiar with the need, when dealing with skin conditions, to formulate products to get round this defence mechanism by emulsifying together hydrophilic and lipophilic components into colloids in order to get water-soluble components past this water-tight boundary and then subsequently even to affect the cells themselves that are powerfully ring-fenced against intrusion. Closely following the skin as a system that is permanently under external influence and thus risk of attack is the gut, with its selective, yet also highly susceptible, digestive system. The next defence is the aptly named first-pass digestive mechanism designed to metabolise, break-down and render harmless foreign agents. The cells themselves are surrounded by walls of macromolecular proteins with brilliantly devised selective molecular portcullises and drawbridges that have to be bridged in order to deliver medicines at this level.

The difference between a poison and a medicine may often be in the dose but the body's defence systems do not have an ability to distinguish between the benign influence of the physician and an incursive attack.

So medicine has an inbuilt difficulty – how to optimise the dose to have the desired effect without poisoning the patient (iatrogenic disease). This difficulty, the linked issues of formulation and dosage, is as old as medicine itself and is an area that science has always studied. In order to understand the whole problem of getting past the body's defence systems in a predictable and controlled way, pharmacy undergraduates have for many years had to study modules in inter-facial phenomena that underpin colloidal chemistry (Rawlins 1977). Not only are most pharmaceutical delivery systems colloidal but the main biological structures, such as blood, brain and bone, are indeed colloids themselves. The elucidation of this subject leads to the ability of the drug industry to deliver nanoparticles to specific cellular targets.

Evolution as a driver of herbal complexity

Plants too have developed (for a rather longer time than animals) under similar protective constraints as animals, with the one major difference being that most animals can move to optimise their environment, whereas most plants are immobile. This has severe consequences for plant defence mechanisms, although many of the basic biochemical parameters for plants and animals are the same.

Evolution of the patho-physiological activity of herbal medicines did not occur by accident; neither did it arrive by 'design' but more by a combative process in which species have struggled to out-compete each other since the origin of life. Although beneficial mutations may be accidental, taking adaptive advantage of them for successful evolution of species is a 'one-way' and thus, in a sense, a 'purposeful' process. That we find the anti-microbial activity of some plants to be a benefit to us is therefore a happy consequence of the fact that, in order to survive, plant species have needed to develop ways of combating microbial attack – by attacking microbes. The same principles hold true for practically all xenobiological activity. That plants (and sometimes specific plant compounds) can have physiological effects on the mammalian cardiovascular, respiratory, digestive, musculoskeletal, neuro-endocrine systems and so on, is direct testament to the constancy of evolutionary development. The ancestors of every living thing endlessly mutated to re-adapt to the continuous evolution of effective competitive adaptation in a dynamic, interlinked web of ever increasing complexity.

The cells of most of the thousands of medicinal plant parts identified in the world's pharmacopoeia and in the materia medica of herbalists often contain only very small fractions of biopharmaceutically active chemical compounds. Such compounds may be very 'expensive' to the plant to manufacture, in terms of energy or of the genetic sacrifices made during their evolutionary development. As well as to understand their action, coincidentally these help scientists to identify and classify plants (chemotaxonomy). Adaptive processes are required by fundamental laws of competition to optimise these very valuable resources. Such processes may frequently extend to the whole plant tissue and this is sensibly and practicably acknowledged under European law where the 'active ingredient' of a herbal medicine is defined as the whole plant tissue (the 'herbal drug') and not just one or more standardised or purified molecules (Europe 2002).

Stahl (1888) may have been the first to suggest that plants have evolved chemical compounds in order to ward off attack by animals. We now realise that compounds have also been developed during evolution, not only for defence but also to facilitate the extremely complex and inter-related demands of reproduction, shelter, symbiosis and even community structure. For example, Dodson *et al.* (1969), and Brehm and Krell (1975) demonstrated mutualistic interactions between the evolutionary adaptiveness of plants with pollinators and fruit dispersers. Janzen (1973) discussed the 'community structure' of secondary compounds produced within a single plant, pointing out the huge range of possible synergies amongst plant defences. Rhoades and Cates (1976) argued that for plant-herbivore coevolution the most important independent variables are probably spatial and temporal and that the evolution of defensive chemistry is subject to the same general arguments as mechanical and morphological defences. Atsatt and O'Dowd (1976) elaborated a theme that members of plant communities are functionally dependent upon properties of the whole community. Rhoades (1977) outlined a general theory of optimal defence of organisms, suggesting a number of important hypotheses and citing evidence that specialist defences would be most effective against generalist herbivores, which he argued should give rise to a divergent system of chemical defences. In reviewing the biology of plant defences, Janzen (1977) pointed out that plants are collections of 'anachronistic traits that at any given time have caught up with contemporary selective pressures to a highly variable degree'. Brattsten (1979) reviewed the development of physiological defence mechanisms against plant allelochemicals leading to complex 'systems' of biochemical action across whole biological phyla. Many essential metabolic pathways are common to both plants and animals. Others are more specific. Probably more than 40,000 plant secondary metabolites have now been identified (Siegler 1995) and several thousand identifiable chemical species may co-exist within a living plant cell, most of which are protein-based. The endocrine system is a particularly well noted example of the much-conserved common inheritance between plants and animals (Baker 1995, Stoka 1999, Schultz 2002) with evident consequences for the success of endobiogenie (Lapraz 2012).

At the fundamental level of plant chemical defence against predation, for example when an insect munches into a leaf, the plant suffers disruption to its cellular matrix. This generally, although not invariably, involves the ingestion and to some extent digestion, of plant material. This has therefore always been a very critical control point for the evolution of defences by plants. It therefore seems useful to look at the biological mechanisms that are unlocked when whole plant tissues are disrupted, because this disruption also happens under controlled parameters when plants are extracted by the makers of traditional herbal medicines.

Most metabolic processes are controlled by specific enzymatic proteins (Stoka 1999). A number of signalling proteins have been found to have similar origin, structure and chemistry, although very different physiological function, in both plants and animals (Baker 1995). Proteins are chemically simple but structurally very complex. Their principle enzymatic role as described by Dobson (2003) might be summed up as mutable molecular morphology. That is to say they function by twisting and turning (called 'folding') in order to present appropriate reactive groups to the cellular milieu. The physical stability of these delicate molecular juggernauts is dependent on the chemistry of inter-facial phenomena. The evolutionary imperative for optimisation of plant secondary metabolite activity would therefore suggest that the complex chemistry of proteins (also known as 'proteomics') is a significant factor in the physically structured transport of physiological plant substances within other species. The way 'actives' are wrapped in proteomic pastry and presented to human physiology is akin to the way one wraps a pill in a sweet for an animal or flavours a medicine for a child.

From all this it follows that widely successful species at a given point in time, for example current insects and mammals, are both responsible for the development, and have also been the beneficiary, of the evolution of a wide range of plant chemical products. For this to have occurred, plants must have used any and every possible mechanism available in nature to optimise the biological activity of the ecologically 'expensive' active compounds, that they have evolved. In order to optimise the economic 'cost' to plants (in terms of energy expenditure) of the production of secondary metabolites, evolutionary adaptation must always make use of the widest range of ecological, spatial, morphological, physiological, physical and chemical means of delivery. Thus the mechanisms that plants use to present 'active' compounds and the ecological niches in which these are found, may be as significant as the compounds themselves.

It is now widely held that the evolution of plant competitive strategies accounts for the physiological activity of compounds that scientists have classified as 'plant secondary metabolites' and of which great use is made in phytotherapy today. This author (Chenery 2009) has reviewed the physiochemical basis of the mechanisms of physical structural interactions in plant extracts and reports experiments demonstrating the maintenance of colloidal structure from plants – especially fresh plants – that are extracted into tincture (and to lesser extent into tissanes). Indeed, short-chain alcohols (usually ethanol) are commonly used as co-surfactants in the preparation of emulsions and in simple model experiments on microemulsion systems (Everett 1988, Evans and Wennerström 1999, Gelbart *et al.* 1994). A largely polar mixture, ethanol-water solutions, such as tinctures, are thus a relatively non-toxic way of extracting a wide range of bio-molecules from plants in a form in which many components apparently remain, or become, orally bioavailable. Trace-substances also facilitate proteomic surfactance in plant extraction and the importance of these have been reviewed by Eder and Mehnert (1998).

Conclusion

Thus, despite appearances in the textbooks, there is more to the biological activity of herbal medicines than a fortuitous jumble of 'active' chemicals. As Janzen (1979) pointed out, plants are not just collections of Latin binomials. Herbal medicine is much more than that. As well as employing essential chemical entities, xenobiological activity, of which herbal medicine is a good example, is frequently due to the physical structuring of complete complex systems of specialised cellular logistics. The medicinal action of herbs (ie, the quality of their efficacy and safety) may be highly reliant on such complexity, beneath which may lie one of the most significant fundamental differences between synthetic medicines and whole plant extracts.

Evidently more than the sum of their parts, our understanding of the mechanisms of herbal action has possibly barely touched the surface but, while our traditions remain strong and develop, we will remain on the right track.

Acknowledgements

The author wishes to acknowledge the help, assistance and inspiration of many during the compilation of the information given here, including, to mention but a few: Enid Eden (Keys College), the late Hein Zeylstra, Midge Whitelegg and Dave Greenway (UCLAN), Kate Stokes (Rutland Biodynamics Ltd), Jack Woolley (DMU, Leicester), Haijo Knipgenger (Goetheanum, Dornach), Jens Otto (Steiner Project, Arhuus) and Hans Strüh (WALA, Stuttgart).

References

Atstatt, P.R., and O'Dowd, D.J., 1976. Plant defense guilds. *Science*, 193, 24–29.

Baker, M.E., 1995. Endocrine activity of plant derived compounds: an evolutionary perspective. *Proceedings of the society for experimental biology*, 208, 131–138.

Brattsten, L.B., 1979. Biochemical defense mechanisms in herbivores against plant allelochemicals, In: Rosenthal and Janzen, eds. *Herbivores: their interaction with secondary plant metabolites*. New York: Academic Press.

Brem B.G. and Krell, D., 1975 Flavonoid localization in epidermal papillae of flower petals: a specialized adaptation for ultraviolet absorption, *Science*, 190 (4220), 1221-1223.

Chenery, P., 2009. *Plants, colloids and tinctures –nature's pharmaceutics* [online]. Available from http://www.rutlandbio.com/wp-content/uploads/2009/04/plants-colloidstinctures.pdf [Accessed 1 April 2014].

Dobson, C. M., 2003. Protein folding and misfolding. *Nature*, 426, 884–890.

Dodson, C.H., et al., 1969. Biologically active compounds in orchid fragrances. *Science*, 164, 1243–1249.

Eder M., and Mehnert, W., 1998. Bedeutung pflanzlicher begleitstoffe in extrakten. *Pharmazie*, 53 (5), 285–293.

Europe, 2002. *European pharmacopoeia*, fourth edition, inc. supplements 4.1., 4.2., Strasbourg: Council of Europe.

Europe, 2004, Directive 2004/24/EC of the European Parliament and of the Council of 31

March 2004, *Official journal of the European Union* L136 Brussels: Council of the European Union.

ESCOP, 2009. *Monographs, Second Edition, Supplement, European Scientific C*ooperative on Phytotherapy. Exeter: Thieme.

Evans, D. F., and Wennerström, H., 1999. *The colloidal domain: where physics, chemistry and biology meet.* New York: Wiley-VCH.

Everett, D.H., 1988. *Basic principles of colloid science.* London: Royal Society of Chemistry.

Gelbert, M.G., Ben-Shaul, A., and Roux, D., (Eds.), 1994. *Micelles, membranes, microemulsions and monolayers.* New York: Springer-Verlag.

Gilbert, B., and Alves, L.F., 2003. Synergy in plant medicines. *Current medicinal chemistry.* 10, 13–20.

Janzen, D.H., 1973. *The chemical defenses of plants to pathogens and herbivores.* Systematics Association.

Janzen, D.H., 1973. *Comments on host-specificity of tropical herbivores and its relevance to species richness.* Systematics Association, 5, 201–211.

Janzen, D.H., 1977. Evolution of plant chemical defense against herbivores. *In*: Rosenthal, G.A., and Janzen, D.H., eds. *Herbivores: their interaction with secondary plant metabolites.* New York: Academic Press.

Janzen, D.H., 1979. New horizons in the biology of plant defenses. *In*: Rosenthal, G.A., and Janzen, D.H., eds. *Herbivores: their interaction with secondary plant metabolites.* New York: Academic Press.

Lapraz, J.C., and de Clermont-Tonnerrs, M.L., 2012. *La médecine personnalisée* (Sciences Humaines), Paris: Odile Jacob.

Mills, S., and Bone, K., 2000. *Principles and practice of phytotherapy.* Modern HDP, London: Churchill Livingstone.

Mills, S., and Bone, K., 2005. *The essential guide to herbal safety.* St. Louis MI: Elsevier Churchill Livingstone.

HRH The Prince of Wales, Juniper, A., and Skelly, I., 2010. *Harmony – a new way of looking at our world.* London: Harper Collins.

Rawlins, E.A., 1977. *Bentley's textbook of pharmaceutics.* 8th Ed. London: Balliére Tindall.

Rhoades, D.F., and Cates, R.G., 1976. *Recent advances in phytochemistry*, 10, 168–213.

Rhoades, D.F., 1977. In: Rosenthal, G.A., and Janzen, D.H., Eds. *Herbivores: their interaction with secondary plant metabolites.* New York: Academic Press.

Schultz, J.C., 2002. Shared signals and the potential for phylogenentic espionage between plants and animals. *Integrative and computational biology*, 42, 454–462.

Siegler, D.S., 1995. *Plant secondary metabolism.* USA: Kluwer Academic.

Stahl, C.E., 1888. *Pflanzen und schnecken. eine biologische studie über die schutzmittel der pflanzen gegen schneckenfraß.* [Plants and snails, a biological study regarding protection of plants against slugs]. PhD Thesis: Jena.

Stoka, A.M., 1999. Phylogeny and evolution of chemical communication: an endocrine approach. *Journal of molecular endocrinology*, 22, 207–225.

Research informing herbal medicine practice

Julie Whitehouse

The herbal practitioner working in the UK in the twenty first century is facing many challenges unprecedented in the history of Western herbal practice. The context of modern practice is within the field of complementary medicine, and to a great extent relates to the definitions and constraints of the conventional biomedical model and the predominant social and health care systems. Herbal medicine nevertheless still draws strongly on traditional practice and interpretations of the empirical knowledge of the herbs and their uses, and on a range of different philosophies and principles of practice and of patient management and treatment. The challenge for the herbal practitioner today is to create a meaningful synthesis of these traditional approaches with the increasing volume of scientific research and the current knowledge base of clinical medicine.

Most patients' first visit to the practitioner follows a doctor's consultation, often with a diagnosis and orthodox drug treatment. The practitioner is thus required to offer the herbal treatment in the context of shared care, with consideration of the consequences of combining concurrent treatments and the need to communicate with other health professionals. It is increasingly rare that herbal medicine can be justified as an alternative treatment.

The herbalist operates as an independent practitioner, with treatments based on the individual assessment of the patient following an extensive consultation, considering all factors of wellbeing, health and disease. Aims of treatment may not be solely targeted at the presenting condition but have a wider reference to preventative medicine and enhancing health and vitality.

The assessment of the patient is therefore quite subjective and the treatment plan is consequent on the practitioner's experience and individual practice style.

Programmes for initial training and continuing professional development offer a comprehensive and approved curriculum aimed at educating and maintaining the professional practitioner. Professional membership requires the practitioner to conform to agreed standards and regulations to ensure safe and ethical practice. Notably individuals have freedom to adopt and develop their own practice styles and interpretations and practitioners often work with their own preferred herbal combinations and prescriptions. There is undoubtedly considerable variation across the profession and this diversity of Western herbal practice has been little researched. Current research in the University of Westminster herbal research team in this arena includes an ethnographic study of practice and practitioners and patient experiences of consultations and herbal treatment. Some valuable research has been carried out into the patient experience of Western herbal practice giving further insight into the nature of practice (Evans 1993, Little 2006, Nissen 2008, 2010, Nissen and Evans 2012, Stewart 2010), but there is a need for more detailed research in this area.

Important issues arise for the training of herbalists and the role and responsibilities of the herbal educator. The training programme and standards are prescribed by a core curriculum [available on the website of the European Herbal and Traditional Medicine Practitioners' Association (EHTPA)] and the BSc honours degree courses are accredited by the EHTPA Accreditation Board, aiming to standardise training across the profession in the UK. However the educator inevitably must accept a level of responsibility in the teaching and learning experience offered to the students and in shaping and defining our future practitioners. This will strongly influence not only the practice style and approaches at the point of entry into practice but also provide the underpinning knowledge and understanding of future practice development. It might be said that the educator may even more keenly feel the challenges referred to above for the individual practitioner.

The nature of herbal practice has undergone great changes in the last few decades with the promotion of the sciences and evidence-based practice. The education curriculum has a major focus on the health and plant sciences and biomedicine approaches; this is a vital and expanding knowledge base for the student and for the practitioner in continuing professional development. However it is feared that this emphasis may have resulted in an undesirable neglect of traditional herbal philosophies and values and of our extensive materia medica, and a perception that our historical practices developed over centuries are of less value and relevance.

Are we at risk of losing our traditional identity and access to, and use of, many of the herbs which have been much valued for so long? Can we be sure that the evidence-based medicine advocated within modern health professions is the way forward and that it is really meaningful for efficacy and safety of herbal practice? How do we retain the traditional knowledge and skills and reinterpret them into the modern context, and encourage students to respect and preserve our heritage? How best can the science of herbal medicine and current medical understanding and practices be applied to modern herbal practice? Importantly, what can we draw from research findings to update and inform our practice?

The evidence base for herbal medicine is extensive and variable in quality, and is often subject to much criticism in failing to meet the highest standards of evidence in critical review. Cochrane reviews are highly respected as applying rigorous assessment standards to review of clinical trials and only a few of the most researched herbs are positively reviewed (Cochrane Collaboration 2014, Cochrane Systematic Reviews and Protocols 2006). Vital information is often missing, such as product origin and phytochemical profile, details of manufacture or preparation, and problems arise with interpreting multiple herb mixtures and complex interventions and treatment outcomes. Poor study design and small trials result in limited value for the research findings. Gagnicr *et al.* (2006a, 2006b) usefully reviewed evidence of the deficiencies in 206 randomized clinical trials in herbal medicine highlighting incomplete information on the herbal product and poor trial design, and made recommendations for reporting randomised controlled trials of herbal medicine interventions. The problems within the research trials not only reduce their value in contributing to the evidence base, but often result in the findings having little relevance to practice. Clinical trials may be directly relevant only to the selected study group and the methodology used, the preparation and dosage chosen, the length of study, and the selected outcomes measured, which are likely to be very different from the values applied in practice.

The pressure to have a reliable evidence base undoubtedly derives from the wider scientific and health communities and it is a critical issue for the credibility of herbal medicine, clinical surveillance and the regulation of herbal products. The practitioner can indeed draw very important information with respect to the desired herbal quality, the likely mechanism of action, and the value of the treatment for specific pathologies or body systems. The understanding of the aetiology and pathology of disease can be matched to the updated understanding of the herb's phytochemistry and pharmacological actions. Within the context of shared care and concurrent treatments, the practitioner can both maximise the contribution of the herbal treatment and ensure adverse interactions are avoided (Kellermann *et al.* 2011).

There is widespread concern about the effectiveness of antibiotic drugs which is threatened by the development of microbial resistance. The potential for alternative treatment with herbal medicine has been positively reviewed by the EHTPA based on an extensive review of the evidence base (EHTPA 2014, see also the chapter by Michael McIntyre).

The modern practitioner is required to constantly update and integrate into their practice the extensive and changing information on herbs from a wide range of sources, which demands considerable skills in research and critique.

St John's wort (*Hypericum perforatum* L.) may be used as a notable example of an extensively researched herb that has gained approval in the evidence based assessment process. This research is valuable in offering the practitioner a greater understanding of the herb's pharmacological activity on brain receptor sites influencing mood and depression, but also highlights its action on liver enzymes. The practitioner must consider the consequences of combining the herb with psychoactive drugs sharing similar pharmacological mechanisms. Much importance is placed on the likelihood of increased clearance of drugs via the liver and the undesirability of combination with a wide range of medicines (Linde *et al.* 2008).

Phytochemists and pharmacologists have offered much to the understanding of the herbs and their constituents, defining typical phytochemicals of the herbal species and allowing authentication with expected levels for good-quality extracts and ensured pharmacological actions (Liu 2011). As much of this research is based on single chemical extracts, *in vitro* cytology studies and animal trials, there must be some caution in relating it to practical applications.

The likely actions of a herb which has had little investigation may reasonably be inferred from the research evidence of another herb with similar constituents, although it is not necessarily dependable to predict the actions of a whole herb based on its phytochemicals. The much researched baical skullcap (*Scutellaria baicalensis* Georgi) popular in Chinese medicine has a similar phytochemical profile to our Western favourite, skullcap (*Scutellaria lateriflora* L.), lending evidence to support the therapeutic potential of the latter little researched herb (Brock *et al.* 2013).

A single herb can be seen to have multiple active constituents and pharmacological actions and whole-herb preparations are often seen to be superior to isolated extracts of single constituents (Williamson 2001). Turmeric (*Curcuma longa* L.), ideally illustrates the capacity for multiple pharmacological activities in a single herb with demonstrated antioxidant, antineoplastic, antiviral, anti-inflammatory, antibacterial, antifungal, antidiabetic, anticoagulant, cardiovascular protective, hepatoprotective, and immunostimulant actions (Kumar and Sakhya 2013).

Just as it is difficult to analyse the pharmacological actions of the complex constituents of a single herb, it is even more complex to predict the synergistic interactions in the mixed-herb preparations favoured by practitioners. The benefits of synergy in complex herbal preparations and the complications of assessing their potential has been addressed by a number of authors (Spinella 2002, Wang and Xia 2012, Williamson 2001).

The research on some of our most important herbs may reassuringly confirm traditional use or reveal new efficacies, but unfortunately this does not extend to the majority of the herbs within our materia medica; we can only apply traditional or empirical knowledge to many of our most valued traditional and little researched herbs. It can be argued that the most important thing to know about a herb for the practitioner is how to select, prepare and apply it with the best outcomes for the patient's resolution of the disease state. Practitioners may reflect on how much they rely on their experience of using a herb compared to its evidence base or lack of it.

The extensive records contained in Herbals and the writings of herbalists through the ages provide an invaluable resource for the practitioner. Tobyn *et al.* (2012) give an excellent presentation of the challenges of researching traditional writings and interpretations into the modern context. It is often possible to trace the reiteration of information through time and from different authors and sources, with inaccuracies and modifications accumulating to give a much distorted picture. It must be argued that the therapeutic properties of some herbs which were valued as the best treatments of their time may have little relevance in the modern materia medica; some herbs are inevitably rejected now due to their undesirable toxicity or adverse reactions, or even just to limited evidence of efficacy.

In recent years access to a number of herbs has been lost to herbal practice following concerns about safety and adverse reactions. The decisions leading to the banning of herbs are complex and not based solely on assessment of scientific evidence and clinical risk. Decisions are often dependent on complex and debatable interpretations of data and involve dominant social and political factors, with different national regulations governing botanical medicines. The case of kava kava (*Piper mythisticum* G. Forst) illustrates the diversity and complexity in regulation of herbal products (WHO 2007). Kava undoubtedly suffered from a dramatic rise in popularity as an anti-anxiety remedy with huge increases in over the counter sales in the Western world, but it was subsequently banned in many places due to adverse reports of liver toxicity, even in the light of uncertainty in the risk assessment. Baker (2011) presents the evidence and considers the different interpretations of the data by scientists, clinicians and regulatory officials. This case highlights the changing context of herbal medicine and some of the risk factors for continued use of the traditional materia medica. The use of herbal medicines is predominantly in over the counter or internet sales, without the assessment by a professional herbalist, and is likely to result in both inappropriate use and failure to detect adverse reactions at an early stage.

The professional herbalist can be seen to be in an often challenging position as herbal practice continues to develop, integrating traditional and ancient medicine with modern scientific and evidence-based practice; all the while having to reconcile often incomplete and conflicting sources of evidence. The increasing level of clinical surveillance and regulatory frameworks makes further demands on the herbal profession to justify their practice and defend their herbal heritage and tradition. Quality assurance of the herbal medicines themselves is crucial and must have a high priority even though resources for research in this area are limited. Perhaps one of the greatest threats derives from poor quality raw herb materials, lack of authentication and overuse of wild or endangered species.

The twenty first century has already seen very significant advances in the development of the profession and the associated manufacturing industry and herbal medicine continues to be a popular and sought after complementary and alternative therapy. The modern herbalist deserves to be recognised as a highly trained and skilled professional, with an important role in offering effective healthcare choices to the public. The profession will benefit from a higher public profile to promote awareness of the herbal practitioner's training and expertise and their role in promoting healthcare and contribution to disease prevention and treatment. Provided there is further investment in research, herbal medicine and its herbs may also prove to have an important role in development of innovative approaches to treatment of a wide range of health problems.

References

Baker J.D., 2011. Tradition and toxicity: evidential cultures in the kava safety debate. *Social studies of science*, 41, 361.

Brock, C., *et al.*, 2013. Identity issues surrounding American skullcap (*Scutellaria lateriflora*) and an optimised high performance liquid chromatography method to authenticate commercially available products. *Journal of herbal medicine*, 3(2), 57–64.

Brock, C., *et al.*, 2013. American skullcap (*Scutellaria lateriflora*): a randomised, double-blind placebo-controlled crossover study of its effects on mood in healthy volunteers. *Phytotherapy research*, DOI, 10.1002/ptr.5044.

Cochrane Collaboration., 2014. Available from: *www.cochrane.org* [Accessed 15 May 2014].

Cochrane Systematic Reviews and Protocols, 2006. *The Cochrane Library*. Available from www.thecochranelibrary.com [Accessed 15 May 2014].

Davidson, E., *et al.*, 2013. Best available evidence in Cochrane reviews on herbal medicine, evidence-based complementary and alternative medicine [online]. Article ID 163412, Available from: http://dx.doi.org/10.1155/2013/163412.

Evans, M., 1993. Herbal medicine expectations and outcome. *British journal of phytotherapy*, 3(2), 81–5.

Evans, S., 2008. Changing the knowledge base in Western herbal medicine. *Social science and medicine* [online]. 68, 2098–2106. Available from: http://www.sciencedirect.com [Accessed 16 May 2014].

European Herbal and Traditional Medicine Practitioners Association, 2014. *EHTPA Accreditation* [online]. Available from: www.ehtpa.eu/standards/accreditation/ [Accessed 17 May 2014].

Gagnier, J.J., *et al.*, 2006a. Quality of reporting of randomized controlled trials of herbal medicine interventions. *American journal of medicine*, 119 (9), 800.e1–11.

Gagnier, J.J., *et al.*, 2006b. Improving the quality of reporting of randomized controlled trials evaluating herbal interventions: implementing the CONSORT statement [corrected]. *Explore (NY)*, 2 (2), 143–9.

Kellermann, A.J., 2011. Risk of bleeding after therapy with standardised *Ginkgo biloba* extracts: systematic review. *International journal of clinical pharmacy*, 33(2), 347–8.

Kumar, N., and Sakhya, S.K., 2013. Ethnopharmacological properties of *Curcuma longa*: a review. *International journal of pharmaceutical sciences and research*, 4(1), 103.

Linde, K., Berner, M.M., and Kriston, L., 2008. St John's wort for major depression [online]. *Cochrane Database of Systematic Reviews*, No. 4, Article ID CD000448. Available from: http://sss.sagepub.com/content/41/3/361 [Accessed 15 May 2014].

Little, C., 2006. Searching for effective health care: a hermeneutic study of traditional herbalism in contemporary British health care [PhD thesis]. University of Southampton.

Little, C.V., 2009. Simply because it works better: exploring motives for the use of medical herbalism in contemporary UK health care. *Complementary therapies in medicine*, 17, 300–308.

Liu, W.J.H., 2011. *Traditional herbal medicine research methods: identification, analysis, bioassay, and pharmaceutical and clinical studies.* Hoboken: Wiley-Blackwell.

McMullen, M.K., *et al.*, 2014. The effects of herbal bitters, *Gentiana lutea* and *Artemisia absinthium*, and of coffee and caffeine on digestive and cardiovascular physiology. *Journal of ethnopharmacology*, article in press.

Nissen, N., 2008. Herbal healthcare and processes of change: an ethnographic study of contemporary women's practice and use of Western herbal medicine in the UK: Unpublished PhD Thesis. The Open University. Milton Keynes. UK.

Nissen, N., (2010). Practitioners of Western herbal medicine and their practice in the UK: beginning to sketch the profession. *Complementary therapies in clinical practice*, 16, 181–186.

Nissen, N., and Evans, S., 2012. Exploring the practice and use of Western herbal medicine: perspectives from the social science literature [online]. *Journal of herbal medicine*, 2, 6–15. Available from: http://www.sciencedirect.com [Accessed 15 May 2014].

Spinella, M., 2002. The importance of pharmacological synergy in psychoactive herbal medicines. *Alternative medicine review*, 7 (2), 130–137.

Stewart, C., 2010. Hermeneutical phenomenology: girls with Asperger's syndrome and anxiety and Western herbal medicine [online]. Available from: <http://researchrepository.napier.ac.uk/4486/1/Published_Thesis_version_z_June_2011.pdf [Accessed 4 June 2013].

Tobyn, G., Denham, A., and Whitelegg, M., 2011. *The Western herbal tradition, 2000 years of medicinal plant knowledge*. London: Churchill Livingstone, Elsevier.

Wang, X., *et al.*, 2012. A systems biology approach to uncovering pharmacological synergy in herbal medicines with applications to cardiovascular disease. *Evidence-based complementary and alternative medicine*, 2012: Article ID: 519031.

Williamson, E.M., 2001. Synergy and other interactions in phytomedicines. *Phytomedicine*, 8 (5), 401–409.

World Health Organization, 2007. *Assessment of the risk of hepatotoxicity with kava products*. Geneva: WHO.

Learning from plants

Keith Robertson

Introduction

As traditional herbalists we have inherited a rich garden of knowledge about medicinal plants from our forebears and when asked, many indigenous cultures refer to their herbal pharmacopoeia as being revealed to them by the plants themselves. Standing almost diametrically opposed to this sort of intuitive and empirical wisdom, is the reductionist scientific model of investigation which forms the basis of modern orthodox medicine. At present, the latter always has to involve the use of animal experiments at some stage in its development before new drugs can be tested on humans. The idea of trying to alleviate suffering in one part of creation by causing it in another is seen by many as deeply flawed. Also problematic is the question of whether herbalists should adopt this route as a valid scientific methodology, given that this approach has already caused much suffering in humans: a number of drugs fully tested under these conditions then went on to cause major damage. There are major forces at play here, but given the choice what should the future of appropriate herbal research look like? This article explores the options open to us and endeavours to remind us that, as the plants are doing the main work should we not somehow be consulting them?

Herbal medicine vs. Herbal medication

As a profession, we have explored the ways in which we are similar to conventional medicine and yet our client base is often loyal to us because they perceive we are different. It is important to celebrate our differences for a number of crucial reasons. There is the hope, especially amongst our more recent graduates, that herbal medicine will be accepted into the National Health Service (NHS) but Barker (2007) makes an important distinction between herbal medicine – a holistic, practitioner-led discipline and herbal medication – an over the counter product that can often bear little resemblance to the original plant. The herbs as medication may well enter main-stream medicine, for example in Germany in 1993, more than 5 million prescriptions were written for ginkgo (*Ginkgo biloba* L.) with sales amounting to US$280 million (Brown 1996) although this was sold as a standardised extract rather than the whole herb.

However, if herbs are merely phytopharmaceutical agents and they are asked into mainstream medicine why would they need to take a herbalist along with them? Surely it would make more sense to ascertain the pharmacologically active ingredients, purify or synthesise the compounds, test in animals followed by clinical trials and then doctors could prescribe the drugs for us? Of course, if this approach worked as well as reductionist science says it should herbalists would all be out of a job! So it is hugely important for our continued future, regardless of what happens in the NHS, to develop and celebrate how we are different in our approach to diagnosis and prescribing whilst maintaining public safety.

We have a duty to our patients to preserve an effective alternative to conventional medicine for a number of reasons, not least because despite some impressive short-term successes, in the main biomedicine does not seem to work that well. Figures for the US show that medical care is now one of the most common causes of death after heart disease and cancer; accounting in 2000 for 225,400 deaths of which 106,000 were due to adverse drug effects. This is just the number of patient deaths on prescribed drugs and does not include adverse drug events which are labelled possible or a further 7,400 deaths due to medical errors (Starfield 2000). Within three years the death toll had climbed to 300,000 (Null 2003). It all helps to put our herbal endeavours and safety record into perspective. Plants and animals co-evolved and the whole reductionist paradigm cuts across all this.

Another huge problem is the corruption that has been allowed to build up in the dynamic between the powerful vested interests within modern mainstream medicine. A shocking example of this came to light in 2010 when the drug company AstraZeneca was fined US$520 million for the 'off label', or unapproved, marketing of Seroquel. Approved only for the short-term treatment of schizophrenia and acute bi-polar disorder, AstraZeneca had for five years been aggressively marketing it as a long-term cure-all in elderly patients and children; even though clinical studies had shown serious and debilitating side effects, particularly in these groups (Stier 2010). The same company was fined US$355 million for fraudulently marketing their prostate cancer drug Zoladex in 2003, so these vast fines seem to have not deterred them from their nefarious practices. Small wonder when you consider these fines represented only about 20 per cent of the profits they made in the process. By settling out of court there were no convictions, no one went to jail and the fines were treated simply as a cost of doing business (Stier 2010).

Drug companies in the US in the period from 1998 and 2004 spent over US$900 million in lobbying on at least 1,600 pieces of legislation including US$90 million on election campaigns. (Sheldrake 2013). Hardly an even playing field for the rest of us and the patients concerned.

Before you say it couldn't happen here in the UK (for the moment AstraZeneca is a UK company) it is worth remembering that the Medicines and Healthcare Products Agency (MHRA) is funded by the pharmaceutical industry. For example in 2008 the MHRA decided that a new warning about side effects should appear on the label of statins but the industry managed to deprive the 4 million people on this prescription of this information for a sickening 21 months because they did not agree with the wording (Goldacre 2009)! Governments and regulatory bodies are meant to curb such abuses but how effective are they? Even more recently the Tamiflu vaccine scandal revealed that we spent nearly £500 million on stock-piling a drug that was no better that paracetamol in the treatment of bird flu; the research on which was available but was intentionally suppressed for private gain at the expense of public good. The scariest thing about this is that no law was broken by the company Roche (Goldacre 2014). What worries me most about the system is that somewhere there are researchers who were aware of this and yet said nothing. We can sympathise with the uncomfortable position of a potential whistle-blower, but we can in no way condone their lack of action or the actions of the company executives who are prepared to intentionally harm people for profit. So doctors it seems are between a rock and a hard place; on the one hand a demotivated public and on the other, an aggressive drug industry. Modern drug therapies are mainly based on herbs, some 70 per cent derived from them. If we want to rescue our herbs from such dubious practices what are the alternatives?

Approaches to herbal medicine research

The gold standard of randomised, controlled, double blinded placebo trials (RCTs) are based on the model of viewing herbs as pharmacological agents only and removing the practitioner/observer from the therapeutic effect thus producing quantifiable, reproducible and statistically significant data but for herbal medication alone (Lewith *et al.* 2003). The synergistic interactions of constituents within a herb itself as well as combined within a prescription and the importance of the therapeutic relationship between patient-practitioner and plant as experienced in herbal practice are not considered in this type of trial. This is swimming against the tide of our co-evolutionary history with plants as food and plants as healing agents. This is not to say that herbalists are unable to conduct RCTs but surely only if the experience of the patient on the trial mirrors that of an individual consultation, can such trials inform herbal practice. For example the treatment of menopausal symptoms by qualified herbal practitioners (Green *et al.* 2007) and the effect of herbal relief in chronic pain (Mills *et al.* 1996). This so called black box approach to RCTs is a more realistic framework to represent what actually goes on in herbal practice (St George 2001).

The majority of herbal research available in the literature is limited in terms of informing professional herbal practice. This is for a variety of reasons: most research is conducted by non-herbal practitioners (Lecrubier *et al.* 2002) and adopting the same preparation, same dose, same duration of treatment approach in non-herbalist led clinical trials does not concur with the individual tailor-made treatment plan and variable prescribing witnessed in professional herbal practice. Many laboratory based projects use isolated constituents of a herb (Weiss 1988) and sometimes, the wrong species and part of plant are used and even non-traditional therapeutic use applied (Taylor *et al.* 2003). Focusing on herbs as pharmacological agents does not consider the energetic, synergistic and traditional uses (Wood 2004).

A much better model was the trial undertaken by Bensoussan *et al.* (1998), who compared individualised treatment with a herbal consultation to standard formula treatment and found that the individualised treatment maintained longer-lasting positive effects for patients after they had discontinued the treatment than the non-individualised treatment. Given the preceding arguments, it is clear that the herbal medicine profession needs to develop its own paradigm of holistic and practitioner relevant research and not blindly adopt what has gone before.

The Scottish School of Herbal Medicine (SSHM) was set up in 1992 as an independent charity to promote holistic research and education, although the innovative research programme ceased in 2010 due to the economic crisis and a lack of external funding. The main research initiatives that we explored were Goethean or holistic science (Robertson 2003), case studies and case series research (Wood 2006, Robertson and Robertson 2009). One of our greatest strengths as herbalists is in our individually tailored approach and herbalists would do well to collate their case studies and start to replicate the huge empirical data base of disciplines such as Traditional Chinese Medicine (TCM). Goethean or holistic science fitted in with the SSHM ethos of being cruelty free, sustainable and relevant to herbal practitioners and because the other danger is that we could follow conventional medicine in its reductionist paradigm just as it is starting to emerge from this. Mind-body medicine has recently enjoyed much more mainstream attention with the development of psychoneuroimmunology. On one level it seems obvious to say that the mind controls the body but the full ramifications of this are far reaching. It is fascinating to think that our minds and therefore our beliefs create our world. A simple example of this is the effect of our emotions, for example, if we get angry we create stress hormones and so our anger becomes manifest in the physical world. Lipton (2008) in his seminal work, *The Biology of Belief*, has importantly moved the main control centre of the cell from the nucleus to the cell membrane. This is where the cell interacts with its surroundings and stresses the crucial importance of the environment in the cell's life. This interchange has recently even been shown to allow the cell to change its own genetic code in response to environmental conditions (Lipton 2008).

The Human Genome Project (HGP) made a basic assumption that the more complex an organism was the greater the number of genes it would possess. Given that bacteria have between 3,000 and 5,000 genes and a simple roundworm around 23,000 genes, the considerably more complex fruit fly was found to have only 18,000 genes. When the project was completed at a cost of some US$3 billion it was found that humans have only 23,000 genes, almost the same number as the humble roundworm (Lipton and Bhaerman 2012).

Evolutionary understanding

Biotechnology companies had hoped to reap huge benefits from the HGP but lost an estimated US$40 billion in the process. Even a simple sea urchin has more genes than a human at 26,000 and many animals and plants have more genes than us, with rice having 38,000 genes (Sheldrake 2013). Billions have been spent to confirm that the most important factors for human health are diet (e.g. the recently announced 10 pieces of veg and fruit a day) and lifestyle, exercise and of course our mental attitude to life. Herbalists could have produced these conclusions for free and spent the money more wisely elsewhere, in holistic education and research. However, perhaps the money was well spent if it teaches humanity a bit of humility.

Intuitively I have always believed that evolution is purposeful and the idea of the human beings 'pulling' the course of evolution towards them is an attractive concept. Recent developments in biology and physics are starting to support this position (Lipton 2008). An important part of evolutionary theory has oscillated between opposing poles since before Darwin's day. The debate was about whether characteristics acquired during an organism's lifetime could be inherited by its offspring. Jean-Baptiste Lamarck's theory of evolution (Sheldrake 2013) which predated Darwin's by more than 50 years, had this concept at its core. Lamarck's most famous example was the giraffe, whose long neck he proposed was acquired by stretching up to eat leaves over generations. Darwin essentially concurred. With the rise of the gene theory of life this became a heresy and Neo-Darwinism held sway for most of the twentieth century and evolution was seen as a random purposeless process that organisms initially played no active part in. Lamarck and his ideas fell into disgrace. However the beginning of this century has seen the pendulum swing the other way again, with the growing acceptance that some acquired characteristics can indeed be inherited. This new science is called epigenetics, the pre-fix epi signifying over or above genetics. Conventional science's view has been that the process was entirely random (Sheldrake 2013).

However, in 1998 John Cairns a prominent geneticist published an interesting experiment. He chose bacteria which could not digest lactose and put them into cultures whose only available nutrient was lactose. The predicted result was quite straightforward – they would die. However, surprisingly they thrived. The only way they could do this was to have purposefully mutated their own genes that dealt with lactose metabolism. Cairns findings were greeted by the journal *Science* in an editorial entitled *A heresy in evolutionary biology*. However, widespread repetition of Cairns' experiment has led to the gradual acceptance of the importance of epigenetics (Sheldrake 2013). What this confirms is something that herbalists have always appreciated: that it is the environment, or rather our perception of the environment that is critical for our well-being.

If epigenetics is the new biology the new physics is quantum physics which came about partly because, just as we had become comfortable with the fact that light moves in waves, there came the realisation that it could also exist as a particle. Quantum physics crucially also introduced us to what a key role the observer plays in any experiment. Light and indeed all matter in effect, exists as a possibility in wave or pure energy form and the observer collapses that possibility into a particle with the act of observation (Samanta-Laughton 2006). A good analogy here would be to consider the dynamic between a dancer and the dance. When we observe a dance, what are we seeing? Are we seeing the dancer or the dance? One cannot exist without the other and in some ways they are two different things; another dancer could of course do the same dance. And so there is a duality here but in terms of human sensibility there is also a unity. The universe seems to exist as a possibility until we, as observers, collapse it down into our experience of reality. If all this sounds a bit fanciful we have to remember that quantum mechanics has given us modern technologies that are now commonplace for example, the computer, mobile phone and more recently, CAT scans. As modern physicists talk more and more like eastern mystics, there is a feeling of a circle closing (Samanta-Laughton 2006).

Modern medicine with its heavy focus on drugs is yet to really embrace the possibilities inherent here but perhaps herbalists and our centuries of connection to medicinal plants have always exploited this special flow of information. Central to quantum theory is the concept of the quantum vacuum or the Dirac Sea; or as I prefer to call it, inspired by Patti Smith's song, 'Horses', the sea of possibilities. The universe, it appears, is information rich and we and every particle of the universe are bathed in the same information as we swim together in this sea of possibilities. Physicists and mystics agree - all life is one and every part of the universe is connected, as information is exchanged instantaneously between every part, blowing apart the idea that the speed of light is the fastest speed in the universe. Einstein famously demonstrated that matter is in fact energy in his famous E = MC2. Matter is in effect energy expressing itself and in the beautiful circle of observer and the observed, the universe is here because we are here to see it and we are here because the universe wants to be seen. It has been said that a physicist is an atom's way of expressing itself; is by extension a herbalist a herb's way of expressing itself?

Study the phenomenon not the theory

I have spent a lifetime studying plants and their medicinal virtues through the conventional routes of pharmacology and materia medica but also through contemplative techniques as suggested by the great natural scientist, Johann von Goethe. Goethe was a contemporary of Newton and suggested an alternative science that was wholly embedded in studying the phenomenon as a counterpoint to the growing importance of theoretical science, where the theory becomes more important than the observed object. Science was to become dogma free but of course, as the physicist, David Bohm (1985) suggests, this is of course, pure dogma. Quantum physics shows us that the act of observation changes the phenomenon. Holistic science is therefore an attempt to reunite what has become separated and to honour both the subjective and the objective in the world around us. Conventional science stops the dance and dissects the dancer in the hope of discovering the meaning of the dance whereas holistic science works from the other end by intimately and respectfully observing the dance as a whole and then fully immersed in the phenomenon, only then seeks to find the meaning in the dance. In order to truly see something we need to take it into ourselves and develop our inner and outer perception. Natural objects, Goethe wrote 'should be sought and investigated as they are and not to suit observers but respectfully as if they were divine beings' (Goethe1971 p. 57). Conventional science has spent many years developing more and more complex instruments to measure nature. Goethe (1994, p. 311) suggested an approach to develop the scientists themselves. It was his opinion that 'the human being to the extent that we make sound use of our senses, is the most exact physical apparatus that can exist'. He talked of the need for a 'delicate empiricism which makes itself utterly identical with the object, thereby becoming true theory' (p. 307) and cautioned 'How difficult it is... to refrain from replacing the thing with its sign, to keep the object alive before us instead of killing it with the word' (p. 275).

Therefore, we can study plants by killing them and analysing their phytopharmaceutical entrails or we can take the lead from the new biology and the new physics and accept that all parts of creation are indeed one and are all immersed in the same sea of possibilities. We can strive to study not so much the plant that is visible in the external world but the plant that exists within us. In the end, we probably need both. The modern world requires that we embrace both the particle and the wave.

When Descartes severed the body from the mind, he maintained that animals were merely mechanical devices and that their cries of pain were merely the 'creaking of the wheels' (quoted in Sheldrake 2013) and so vivisection was born and Descartes' followers were encouraged to kick their dogs. This attitude has become entrenched, even up to the present day with Richard Dawkins (1989) suggesting that human beings are 'merely lumbering robots'. As these robots, we are merely the vehicles by which Dawkins' selfish genes travel across the Earth. Dawkins rails against such sins as anthropomorphism and yet has labelled our genes as selfish; this may well be but I prefer to see my own genes as being generous for they have provided me with the opportunity of experiencing this marvellous creation.

If we merely see plants as constituents then we are throwing away a huge part of the experience. In one sense the dancer's costume is a minor part of the equation and yet from an aesthetic point of view, it is paramount to the whole experience. Likewise, the dancer's inner emotions are in one sense peripheral to the execution of the dance, but on a deeper level if the dancer is merely thinking of what they will have for their dinner afterwards, the experience for everyone is surely reduced. I would argue therefore, that the plant's external form and inner reality are equally important to consider alongside the constituents of the plant.

In conclusion

Plants are hugely complex entities and, may I even suggest like us, divine beings. We can see them simply as unconscious individuals or we can try and comprehend the idea of the plant as a member of a wider species, which interconnects with plants both past and future as expressed in the ancient idea of the plant Deva. Physicists have recently discovered that the visible universe accounts for only four per cent of the actual universe; the rest is made up of what they have termed dark matter and dark energy (Samanta-Laughton 2006). The darkness comes from their position of viewing the universe as essentially dead and mechanical. I would like to propose an alternative view which is to see this amazing conundrum, that 96 per cent of our universe is missing, as more evidence of the existence of the life force and to see plants and ourselves as living expression of that life force. To see humans and plants both emerging from the sea of possibilities, separate and yet intimately interconnected. As a profession herbalists have the choice to follow conventional science in the hope that we receive acceptance from the orthodox community or we can stand up and recognise our rich history of holistic investigation and reclaim our birthright as alternative practitioners.

Epigenetics has shown that the genes themselves are less important than the mechanism which switches them on and off. In effect that which makes us unique beings, our individual life force, is not a physical force which is contained in our DNA but a cosmic idea of us which is non-physical and resides elsewhere. Rupert Sheldrake has proposed the concept of morphic resonance and morphic fields to explain the deep connections between all parts of nature. His research is full of stories of pets finding their owners, sometimes thousands of miles away, with no possible explanation other than an unseen connection between them (Sheldrake 2013). I would propose that we should be looking for the same deep connection with our plants. Seeing ourselves as part of the wholeness of the universe rather than distinct from it, gives us a unique opportunity to build a personal relationship with all of our medicinal plants themselves rather than their individual parts. This is no easy endeavour but for the future of holistic herbal healthcare it is something that we need to fully embrace. As Albert Einstein said, "The most beautiful and profound emotion we can experience is the sensation of the mystical. It is the power of all true science."

References

Barker, J., 2007. *History, philosophy and medicine – phytotherapy in context.* West Wickham: Winter Press.

Bensoussan, A., *et al.*, 1998. The treatment of irritable bowel syndrome with Chinese herbal medicine. *Journal of American Medical Association, 280, 1585-1589.*

Bohm, D., 1985. *Wholeness and the implicate order.* London: Routledge.

Brown, D.J., 1996. Phytotherapy - herbal medicine meets clinical science. *NARD Journal*, Vol 3, 41-52.

Dawkins, R., 1989. *The selfish gene.* Oxford University Press.

von Goethe, J.W., 1971. *Goethe's colour theory.* New York: Van Nostrand-Reinhold.

von Goethe, J.W., 1994. *Scientific Studies.* Princetown University Press.

Goldacre, B., 2009. *Dithering over statins; side effects label finally ends.* Available at http://www.theguardian.com/commentisfree/2009/nov/21/statins-side-effects-ben-goldacre. [Accessed 12 May 2014].

Goldacre, B., 2014. *What the Tamiflu saga tells us about drug trials and big pharma.* [online]. Available from: http://www.theguardian.com/business/2014/apr/10/tamiflu-saga-drug-trials-big-pharma [Accessed 12 May 2014].

Green, J., *et al.*, 2007. Treatment of menopausal symptoms by qualified herbal practitioners: a prospective randomised controlled trial. *Family practice*, 24(5), 468-474.

Lecrubier, Y., *et al.*, 2002. Efficacy of St John's Wort extract WS 5570 in major depression: a double-blind, placebo-controlled trial. *American journal of psychiatry*, 159 (8), 1361-1366.

Lewith G., Jonas, W. and Wallach, H., eds., 2003. *Clinical Research in complementary therapies: principles, problems and solutions.* UK: Churchill Livingston.

Lipton, B., 2008. *The biology of belief.* London: Hay House.

Lipton, B. and Bhaerman, S., 2012. *Spontaneous evolution.* London: Hay House.

Mills, S., *et al.*, 1996. Effect of a proprietary herbal medicine on the relief of chronic arthritic pain: a double-blind study. *British journal of rheumatology*, 35, 874-878.

Null, G., 2003. *Death by medicine.* New York: Nutritional Institute of America.

Robertson, K., 2003. *The evaluation of Goethean Science as a methodology for the investigation of medicinal plant properties with specific reference to hawthorn (Crataegus* Spp.*).* Dissertation (MSc). Scottish School of Herbal Medicine. [online] Available from: http//www.veganherbal.com [Accessed 12 May 2014].

Robertson, M. and Robertson K., 2009. The case for case history research. *Scottish Journal of Herbal Medicine*, 1, 51-55. [online] Available from: http://www.veganherbal.com/ library [Accessed 12 May 2014].

Samanta-Laughton, M., 2006. *Punk science: inside the mind of God.* UK: Iff Books.

Sheldrake, R., 2013. *The science delusion.* London: Coronet Books.

Starfield, B., 2000. Is US health really the best in the world? *Journal of the American Medical Association*, 284, 483-458.

Stier, K., 2010. *Curbing drug company abuses, are fines enough?* [online] Available from: http://www.time.com/time/business/article [Accessed 12 May 2014].

St George, D., 2001. Letters to the editor. *Journal of alternative and complementary medicine*, 7 (3), 219-228.

Taylor, J.A., *et al..*, 2003. Effect of oral administration of freshly pressed juice of *Echinacea purpurea* on the number of various subpopulations of B- and T-lymphocytes in healthy volunteers: results of a double-blind, placebo-controlled cross-over study. *Journal of the American Medical Association*, 290 (21), 2824-2829.

Weiss, R.F., 1988. *Herbal medicine.* Beaconsfield Publishing.

Wood, M., 2004.*The practice of traditional Western herbalism.* California: North Atlantic Books.

Wood, M., 2006. *An exploration of the conceptual foundations of Western herbalism and biomedicine with reference to research design.* Dissertation (MSc). *Scottish School of Herbal Medicine.* [online] Available from: http://www.matthewwoodherbs.com/Dissertation.html [Accessed 12 May 2014].

Herbal Experiences

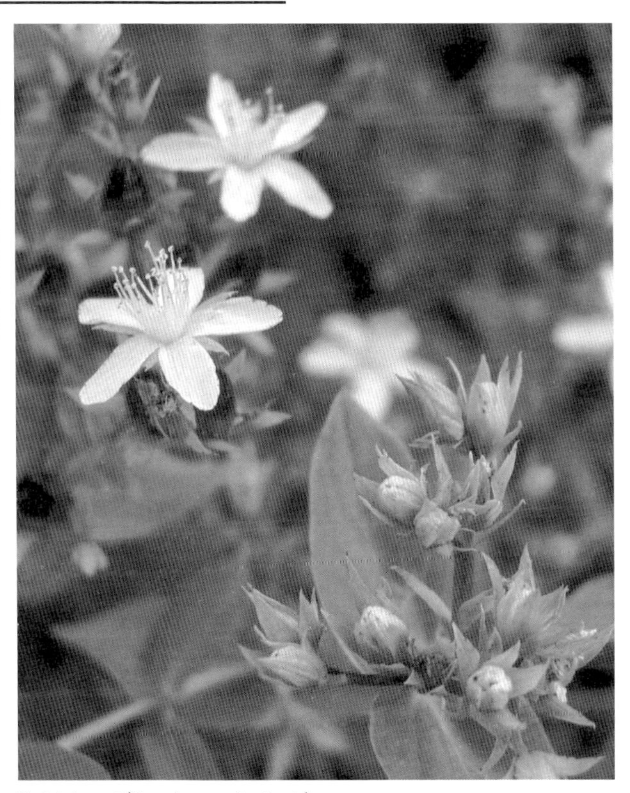

St. John's wort (*Hypericum perforatum* L.)

Practice placements: reflections on herbal consulting rooms I have known

Graeme Tobyn

I registered for training with the School of Herbal Medicine in Tunbridge Wells, Kent after being inspired by Christopher Hedley's course on herbs at the Mary Ward Centre, Queen's Square, Bloomsbury – where herbalists had met at the dawn of the National Association of Medical Herbalists (NAMH). The location for the vast majority of my clinical training was the Balham clinic, a converted Victorian house at the corner of two residential streets in SW12. The clinic was bustling with enthusiastic students and herbalists committed to the furtherance of the profession but the building itself was obviously not purpose-built and it contrasted with two notable external placements during my training: Stephen and Carol Church's well-organised large and welcoming practice room on the ground floor of their home in Coulsdon, Surrey, open to all, and my day with a GP also in Surrey. That day I went with the doctor from a tiny branch surgery where minimal examination took place, to home visits in large houses with offers of wine, then on to the main purpose-built surgery, where with one of the few patients willing to have me in the room, I performed my one and only rectal examination. This was quite a different experience to my Saturdays in Balham.

Stephen Church affirmed that being a herbalist was all about 'tending the shop', in other words being where patients can reach you with certainty at (almost) any time. The GP practice of course must have been established for many years in that town, although the branch surgery looked like a new venture. My own practice, as I will describe it now, has moved more than once and the need to rebuild patient numbers at a new address is much harder than maintaining a base practice where people come to know that you are available, such as my friend and colleague Steve Kippax has done in Suffolk over many years.

I entered practice in London in 1990, briefly in a clinic housed in another Victorian building on Stoke Newington Church Street; then for a happy year behind Islington Green in a small, modern prefab of sorts squeezed in between older buildings on Gaskin Street, N1, which was run by the osteopath Fergal O'Daly, who had once studied with R.D. Laing. The modern setting, more office-like than residential, and good relations with Fergal and other practitioners there who supported the idea of having a herbalist working alongside, I felt contributed to a positive start to my practice. The building now no longer exists.

We then took our growing children out of London to live in better air and attend calmer schools and I set up practice for initially one then two days a week at the Hereford Centre for Natural Health, a very new purpose-built clinic across the Wye from the city centre with ample parking. To each side was a district nurses' office and the local GP surgery; then a dentist and a pharmacy completed the complex. One of the GPs had wanted complementary and alternative medicine (CAM) practitioners alongside; they had formed a charity and raised considerable funds for the building of the 'natural health centre' and their move from an old building in the city centre. I joined them soon after and even worked as practice manager for the charity to supplement my income. The design of the building itself was quirky with compromised head space in the upper floor consulting rooms where I saw patients – it was not suitable for housing the furniture to store my tinctures and dried herbs. But the building itself was modern and felt, as it were, made to hold the practitioners of a future integrated medicine. However, the doctors parted company, a senior partner retired and there was a cultural change in the centre meaning that complementary medicine was no longer offered there. This was the time when a new British Medical Association (BMA) booklet came out with proposals for good working practices with CAM therapists for the benefit of patients. A number of us made a point of informing new patients' GPs, with the patients' permission of course, that they were consulting us. I don't recall ever receiving a reply. I helped a good number of patients suffering with allergies and with 'candida', now called gut dysbiosis, since doctors seemed to be wedded to the older definition of allergy and these 'intolerances' and multi-system presentations did not fit diagnostic taxonomies.

I subsequently expanded into a similar purpose-built complex in Bishop's Cleeve, on the edge of Cheltenham, which was a happier experience than a similar multi-disciplinary practice in Gloucester: this was an extensive prefab, run by a group of acupuncturists whose good practice included sharing case studies – the first steps in developing a common style and breadth of treatment – and they seemed to get the majority of the patients entering the practice doors. In both of the clinics I worked in, other CAM practitioners seemed to recognise the benefits of my herbal training and I helped sometimes with their diagnostic conundrums as much as ideas for remedies.

During this decade, two other opportunities took me into different practice rooms. First I obtained a position as a clinical trainer alongside Sue Hawkey in Bristol on Saturdays in the basement of a building to the side of a grander column-fronted house on a Georgian square in Dowry Square in the Hotwells district. The setting was pleasant and peaceful, with a sense of being hidden partly by the trees in the centre of the square, but the clinic space itself was dark and oppressive, as I recall it. From there the student clinic relocated to the smaller Montpelier Natural Health Clinic in a row of Georgian buildings on Picton Street, Bristol. My drive to Bristol on those Saturdays was down the Wye Valley past Tintern Abbey, which in spring and summer provided a joyous start to the day. We took the students up there one Saturday on a botanising trip. By 1999 Sue Hawkey together with Maggie MacMillan had fitted out the ground floor of a former end terrace in a quiet street in the Larkhall suburb of Bath as a new practice 'Herbs for Health'. There was not only the necessary consulting room and its amenities, but the dispensary was integral to the shop front of the conversion. Sue moved the student training clinic here from Bristol and I shared the supervision with her. Students came from all over the South West. As it had been in Montpelier, the space to accommodate them on the same Saturday in order to provide continuous support and to meet their objective for clinical hours proved a challenge – the shop space was integral to those training days – but the students were very positive and Sue and Maggie had created a very good local presence for the practice.

The second opportunity was to work for a Hereford city centre GP practice. Several CAM therapists were engaged – an acupuncturist, homeopath, osteopath, aromatherapist/reflexologist and myself as herbalist – we enjoyed well-designed and -equipped consulting rooms, computerised GP consultation notes (a beneficial addition to patients' own narratives) and, for me, my usual private charges for the medicines. All the CAM practitioners were asked for referral guidelines and they were often very similar. The GPs of course selected the patients to send through, so the range of conditions seen was different to that in my 'private' practice where anyone failed by the system might come through the door. We seemed to be doing a good job and there was to be an audit of our provision with the possibility of showing value-for-money for our services. The research, however, did not get off the ground before a difficult financial period put an end to our NHS engagement. Nevertheless, I felt that I, like other herbalists, had moved in the course of the decade from old, converted residential houses to accommodation in modern purpose-built clinics or practices with shop fronts. And herbal students were also now being educated on university campuses.

In the new millennium I moved into university education as a senior lecturer on the new BSc in herbal medicine at the University of Central Lancashire. The training clinic situated in the city centre just behind the main street in Preston had been purchased two years earlier. The building was early nineteenth century on two floors with several rooms available for consulting, a generous reception area and a rest room-cum-kitchen. At one point the NIMH library was housed upstairs. There was thus plenty of space but not in the right place; none of the ground floor rooms where patients were seen comfortably accommodated the usual eight students plus herbalist; the building overall was costly to run and required regular repairs. I had the sense of returning to the makeshift Georgian and Victorian buildings! When the course was closed for reasons other than academic ones, the clinic became no longer financially viable and the training for the remaining students was taken in-house. We moved to a well-established multi-disciplinary practice in a spacious Victorian villa in another part of the city run by an osteopath. A compact but efficient dispensary had been designed and fitted out, and patients were seen in a large front room which easily accommodated student groups. The other front room operated as the reception for patients. There was no issue with space here – we even had a break-out room in the practitioners' common room upstairs – and the adjustment was with the clinic's established practitioners who were initially overwhelmed by the influx of students on clinic days! After the student training clinic closed in June 2012, I have continued the practice and to attend to the clinic's patients with herbalist Veda West.

Over this period we have seen support from the doctors' bodies dwindle from recognition that we all need to work together (somehow!) for the benefit of patients to a closing of professional ranks and the rise of supporters of a positivist interpretation of scientific knowledge that excludes herbalists as dangerous meddlers dispensing cocktails of plant chemicals with little idea of what they actually do in the body or how much needs to be given to be effective and safe. We have not been forthcoming with our own studies of what herbalists actually do, how we assess patients and how we decide on what to include in a prescription – we seem always to want to prove that our remedies work rather than study outcomes or patient attitudes and experiences with herbalists.

Fortunately, this situation has changed in the last several years, but there is so much more to do. The closing of most of the university BSc courses after their establishment over 15 years is a worrying development. It is not that our services are needed less – on the contrary, there is more we can contribute to than ever, but we must be very professional in going about it. I have had the opportunity to visit the clinical facilities of other university herbal medicine courses, either through on-site visits as a member of the NIMH Accreditation Board, or as an external clinical examiner or visiting lecturer (I had also worked a few times back in the 1990s as a locum clinician at Middlesex University's Archway Clinic). The training that was valued by my CAM colleagues 20 years ago has been further enhanced in these institutions. Key considerations that are managed with varying degrees of success at such flagship training centres are the provisions for the dispensary and size and facilities of consulting rooms. All the current BSc course dispensaries are large and well-stocked – things have certainly advanced from the spacious cupboards in some of the buildings of old. Good lighting in the consultation rooms for careful examination of the patient is now standard. And to avoid having the patient confront a wall or two of student faces, a live video link arrangement of the kind at the very modern clinical facility on the Lincoln University campus to allow observation from another room is, I think, part of the future direction for training: it is a flexible response to the space issue and allows patients to be seen who might be intimidated by having to share their personal stories with a whole group. If herbal medicine is going mainstream, fewer patients will be of the sort I used to see in multi-disciplinary clinics, who supported alternatives because they believed only in alternatives and could put up with more make-shift arrangements. A patient-centred approach in all aspects is the way forward.

Further Reading

Tobyn, G., 2013. *Culpepper's medicine: a practice of Western Holistic Medicine.* London: Singing Dragon.

Tobyn, G., Denham, A., and Whitelegg, M., 2011. *The Western herbal tradition: 2000 years of medicinal plant knowledge, 1st edition.* Oxford: Churchill Livingston.

My life and work with herbs

Jan de Vries

I have, over the years, seen thousands of patients and received many testimonials, confirming that the herbs have been of great help, where orthodox medicine failed.

As a child I always had a great interest in nature which was probably born in me as both my great grandmother and grandmother were well known herbalists. During the Second World War my mother was asked to go to Arnhem Oosterbeek (in Holland, in the area where 'A Bridge too Far' was filmed) to help out in a home for elderly people. This brought about a turning point in my life as there was no school for me to attend. Next to the house was a large monastery and I became friendly with one of the monks who played a great part in my young life. I must have been intelligent enough to take in what he taught me, much of which made a lasting impression on me. I went to help him in the herb garden every day and he would tell me all about the medicinal uses of the plants, roots and trees. With great passion, the monk taught me the wonders of God's creation in nature.

I still remember how heartbreaking it was when one day my mother said that we had to move, and fast. I have never seen a place empty so quickly as then, which was very sad, but everybody was led to safety. Oosterbeek was bombarded nearly to the ground and the house where we had been living was completely flattened. The death and destruction was overwhelming. With my instilled love for God and Creation, I could not understand why this was happening. I remember that day I promised God that if my mother and I were saved, I would care about the well-being of people for the rest of my life. I hope I have kept that promise in the many years I have devoted to helping people, and I will continue to do so until my dying day!

In 1958 I graduated as a pharmacist. In those days the exams were very difficult, which was emphasized by the fact that only two of us succeeded. I couldn't believe my ears when I was told that I had passed. I arrived back home to be greeted by a local fanfare and was treated like a king. Although my head was bursting with knowledge, I had no idea what the future would hold for me but, with the tremendous welcome I received on returning home, I decided that whatever I did, I would try hard to make a good job of it.

About a year later, I went to a lecture in Amsterdam, where by chance I sat next to the late Alfred Vogel. At that time I did not know who he was, but when he started up a conversation and enthused about his work, I was almost instantaneously converted to his way of thinking. Later, when I told my friends about Dr Vogel, nobody was interested as at that time homeopathy was taboo in Holland. However, the principles of alternative medicine were very attractive to me and, although I lost most of my friends I pursued what was to become my life interest.

I was so fascinated by all Dr Vogel said that I travelled to Switzerland to see what he was doing there and we talked about the prospect of opening the first naturopathic clinic in Holland. As we discussed the future of medicine and health, we came to the conclusion that by making such a clinic accessible to those searching for an alternative approach to orthodox medicine we would be taking a step in the right direction.

During the earlier years, possibly between 1937 -1956 Alfred Vogel carried out a lot of research and development and manufactured the first natural remedies using fresh plants. In 1963 he established Bioforce AG in Switzerland, which is today a leading herbal remedy and food company, operating throughout the world.

When I began working with Dr Vogel, he taught me everything he knew. It was admirable to see how fervently he researched his plants. Dr Vogel carried out his research work mainly with volunteers, his richest source of research was by using patients.

Every plant, flower, root and even the bark of a tree has its own signature and characteristic. When we examine them and learn how they grow, the plants share their knowledge with us. Alfred studied many species to establish whether the signatures of the plants gave an indication about which ailments they might be used to treat. He also needed to guarantee that when prescribing such remedies, there would be no side effects and conducted a lot of research when preparing treatments.

Alfred Vogel and I worked together for nearly 40 years off and on, and although we often went our separate ways, we regularly met up to discuss health issues. I feel privileged that I was the only pupil to whom he taught everything he knew about herbs, health and healthy living. He instilled in me that same great desire to help others and every day I feel proud that I have been able to carry on in his footsteps.

I came to Britain in 1970 and have enjoyed working here with the greatest of pleasure. I began working in Troon, Ayrshire and have established various clinics and Health and Diet Centres throughout the UK.

Herbalism, of course has always been my greatest interest and I was lucky enough to find a herbalist who had been trading in Edinburgh for decades. About 40 years ago I went into the little shop. Although it was not very busy it had a number of customers who went there for remedies and to whom it was a blessing. It had the smell of a real herbal pharmacy and what a delight it was! I immediately felt right at home and started to talk to the herbalist, whose name was John Napier. When I told him I was a pharmacist, he was very interested in my work and also in my interest in herbs. I told him about Dr Vogel, of whom he had heard, and mentioned several others who were in the same profession. We had a great talk. I did not think for one minute that one day I would be the proud owner of that little shop, nor did I realize how much it would come to mean to me in later life.

Many years later I purchased the shop and revitalised the old Napier family philosophies originating from the seventeenth century. Over the years I built up the business and, in 1990, I sold it to Dee Atkinson, a well known herbalist, and the name of Napier's continues to grow and diversify today.

I was also fortunate enough a few years later when I returned to the UK to take over the old herbalist company of Abbott's of Leigh. Mr Abbott left great treasures of prescriptions and very old books that are still of value to me. Together with the Napier's memorabilia and herbal books from Dr Vogel and other herbalists I have inherited, I have a tremendous herbal library of which I am very proud.

I have really enjoyed my years of work in herbal medicine and am still researching. At the moment I am very interested in *Fraxinus americana* L. (white ash). It is a wonderful plant with great possibilities and thanks to the excavations of old mummies, the plant has been preserved for thousands of years and has kept a dead body intact. This tree has also been found in some monastic excavations near Edinburgh. I am currently researching the medicinal properties and hope to document them in the near future.

There is so much work to be done in the field of herbal medicine, and I feel very, very sorry that I have seen in this day and age, that there are so many restrictions now. I am sure that for every illness and disease there is a herb growing out there, in nature, that will be of help to man.

Further Reading

De Vries, J., 2004. *Female cancers: a complementary approach.* Edinburgh: Mainstream Publishing.

De Vries, J., 2001. *The pharmacy guide to herbal remedies.* Edinburgh: Mainstream Publishing.

My encounters with herbal medicine as a patient

Julian Barker

When I arrived in Matron's boudoir with what she explained was a *crise de foie* I did not expect her to reach into her large wooden armoire, draw out a bush of thyme and dismiss me peremptorily with the instruction to infuse it.

The medical orderly came along with several neighbours to see how I was doing, made the infusion and explained that the trigger to the crisis was the notorious *mistral*, the wind that enters through the kidneys and bears down upon the liver, heart and mind, depending upon the disposition of the person and the circumstances in which she or he had been so caught out. Usually *he*, she added, as women are more adept at protecting themselves from this malevolent persecutor, then asked in *patois* about whether an Englishman would know what to do with the rectal thermometer she was brandishing.

The slow and sure healing process provided me with a meditation in which the medicinal plant served as an instructor in a way that the silence of previous mainstream interventions had never hoped to. The term '*crisis of the liver*' does not exist in English culture but then nor do we have a mistral. It is 'the 'flu' we catch and we may also 'have a virus' and 'there is always a lot of it going around'. These and other untestable assumptions suggest a microbial rather than a meteorological assailant. Whatever illness it was that befell this 22-year-old in the south of France, it was certainly calamitous and the strength of taste and smell of the herbal remedy appeared like a manifest ally and gave me the strength to contemplate the pathway that had led me to the crisis. The vigour of the thyme dispelled any sense of baffled victim that I might have entertained and gave me back not only courage and strength but also insight: the calamity that drove the illness had a richer history.

It did not occur to me then that I might become a herbalist although I did envy the herb-sellers at the town's weekly market. Not only the wonderful patter and the amusing, often bawdy, interactions with the passing crowd, but the sheaves of bundled plants, aromatic and beguiling – for this or that ailment – spoke of the surrounding hills, woods and meadows. I had been a student of theatre and would later work in it professionally so these improvised free performances were worthy of study and most entertaining. Years later at the Surrey Agricultural Fair I had a stall of my own, selling not bundles of dried herbs but beautiful living plants in small containers that we had grown at Suffolk Herbs where I had served an apprenticeship. It was exhilarating because the crowd in front of me did not thin from early morning to the sale of the last plant. I had by then done only a couple of years on the tutorial course run by NIMH but that did not prevent me from extolling the virtues of the plants. Working outdoors with the soil certainly seemed healthier than the heated and intense life I had spent as a literary and theatrical agent. From plants in pots, now, to a potted history.

I had left teaching because in the 1960s schools did not pay a living wage; thence, after many adventures, I found myself in an overpaid overexposed position. As my job gave me a free choice of breakfast, lunch and dinner – at the company's expense – I taught myself to cook. I had acquired a luxurious fish kettle from a TV cook and tested it out on a large fish with juniper. The result was enjoyed by everyone except me: I was the only one to become ill, somewhat reminiscent of *crise de foie*. Trying to discern the cause for the upset, I learnt that juniper in excess could harm the kidney. I had lavished the fish with this herb as it reminded me of Juniper Hill, a favourite childhood haunt. I couldn't go into work which at the time meant missing a Sunday evening stint at BBC Television Centre. The following week I had to explain my absence to the floor manager. He fancied himself as an astrologer and told me to avoid not only juniper but also black pepper because subjects with my nativity were constitutionally vulnerable in the kidney.

My professional preoccupations centred around money and the price of reputation and were beset by fear of piracy and poaching. Persuasion and negotiation on behalf of others, whatever the actual merits of the case, had to be pursued to the exclusion of the reasonable, the outcome sealed with watertight contracts, and the buttering of bruised egos. And yet ... I seemed to engage much of the time in finding out what fear, insecurity or vulnerability drove the client's process. As I started clinical training at a NIMH practice in Tunbridge Wells more than a decade later, I had the sense of picking up where I had left off.

At the School of Herbal Medicine, my cohort questioned many things, often to the deep frustration of our teachers but it was not until I had been in practice a while that I realised that we had not always asked the most important question. What was our Theory of Cure? It was a question often put to me by Professor Peter Hylands at Chelsea College where he invited me to talk to his pharmacy students. How did an alterative 'alter vital functions'?

I have in front of me a booklet entitled *Herb Gathering* that was published in wartime by Brome & Schimmer, Botanical Drug Importers, given me by its author Barbara Keen (Keen 1941). Its purpose was urgent: to replace the importation of herbs barred by hostilities with local gathering and drying. The foreword was written by an academic from Oxford Botanic Gardens and begins 'Their possession of healing virtues has always been one of the things that has most interested men and women in plants.' Other contributors come from Kew and the Pharmaceutical Society. The term 'alterative' heads the glossary of medical terms, and Bulletin No. 121 of the Ministry of Agriculture and Fisheries *Medicinal Herbs and Their Cultivation* figures in the short bibliography. Such publications predated the term alternative medicine yet they took for granted what we as student herbalists found difficult to do. Another little book – *In Praise of Wild Herbs: Remedies and Recipes from Old Provence* – lists plants for many ailments from acne to warts by way of prostatitis, shingles and varicose veins. It is a charming book and based upon long practical experience; there is little attempt to divine an organising principle at work. If herbal medicine is a collection of remedies and recipes, do we need, then, merely to learn them by rote and apply them when the case of acne, warts, prostatitis, shingles, varicose veins (or anything between) turns up? The question is partly answered by Ludo Chardenon himself:

> *'...it's a different sort of medicine. You see, from the mechanical point of view, you can take a pill and get an effect – say for constipation. But you will have to keep on taking it, whereas with*

my old decoctions you slowly re-educate the organ which has started to play up and bring it back into phase.' (Chardenon 1985)

At least this tells us that the herb is not simply a remedy for a specific condition. Nonetheless, it fails to emphasise that the medical act precedes the medicinal, that all medical practice is an extension of the impulse to make things better for someone in some sort of trouble. That recourse and the practitioner's response is the primary and necessary act of healing. First comes the request, then the assent and assessment and only then the intervention: medicinal or otherwise. As Avicenna put it more succinctly: '*first the word, then the herb and only then the knife.*' Without understanding fully this truth we herbalists would be little more than purveyors of medicinal remedies.

My second encounter as a patient made this clearer to me: I was diffident in approaching the herbalist as he was one of my teachers and for the reciprocal reason he was with me. He made for me a course of capsules each containing five herbs, one of which was juniper. I am sure that they helped, but I could not smell or taste the plants. The predisposing issues were appropriately addressed but the consultation was rushed on my account and a little awkward. I have since treated students myself and have not done as well for them as my teacher did for me. The assent is not fully symmetrical and, in my case, the journey to the consultation was too small and uncommitted an investment. The outcome of a visit to any herbalist may also depend upon how exasperated you become with a chronic condition and how long you place your own problems behind those of others, from too much stoicism and being too busy. We all need to be sustained: this is part of the purpose of medical practice, but some of us may be resistant to sustenance. I realised then that a successful practitioner needs to be blessed with successful patients: those who have overcome the first hurdle and know how to ask.

Symptomatic medicine has not such a need to ask, for it deals with the present and often with the obvious: one treats a wound when fresh, not one that happened last week. Some remedial medicine is essential: it is tactical: survival may even depend upon it. Aetiological or constitutional medicine, by contrast, is strategic: in trying to modify a structural tendency it seeks connections that have not yet been made and a history that has yet to be uttered. It is founded upon the miraculous fact that each of us started our particular life in our grandmother's womb. The pathway from there to a present dilemma is far from obvious and the unravelling of it will be helped by agents who do not make too loud a noise of their own. Whether we apply ourselves strategically or tactically, herbalists have a rare amount of choice with these our remedies. We are not restricted and confined to problem management as are doctors in mainstream medicine. Most of their interventions *replace* an activity that has been interrupted or compromised: neither prednisolone nor thyroxine usually go by the name of hormone replacement therapy (HRT) but that in effect is what they are. Herbalists sometimes advocate replacement therapy, for instance prescribing progesterone cream derived from *Dioscorea villosa* L. This may be superior to semi-synthetic products but it remains replacement therapy all the same. There may be a place for it but, by analogy with Food Aid, no one doubts the need to feed starving people but, as is often remarked, it is even better to provide them with the means to feed themselves. Too much focus on what is 'missing' from the patient (whether it be micronutrient deficiency or endocrine status) will emphasise the supply side of life at the expense of celebrating the enormous power of humans to extract from their environment and to improvise with what they do have. Away from accident and emergencies and given time, medicinal plants are in the position to support function without the need for replacement.

In contrast to medical practice, I learnt that as a theatrical agent there are five distinct things you could do for the client. Although few could hope to do all five well, you needed to know at which of them you were strongest and which weakest, and never to measure your performance against those who did none of them well. Although the ethos could not be more different, moving from client to patient in my professional life has not seemed entirely discontinuous. Among the myriad of things one may do for a patient, we herbalists have a broader base to sustain in that we tend to be our own pharmacist; and then there may also be botanising, cultivating, collecting and making galenicals.

We must abridge the tales our patients tell us yet how they tell us tells us more than they say. As therapists we need to accommodate wavering and disjointed telling. In other words, the quality of the human attention is the usual conduit for medicine to be successfully introduced and for healing to take place. However, medicinal plants can uniquely provide their own conduit into the lives of our patients: their smell and their taste may feed into the limbic system; they may operate at other levels by way of their touch upon the buccal, oesophageal and later the intestinal mucosae before their constituents fully enter the bloodstream.

I have developed elsewhere this multi-modal hypothesis of graded effects of medicinal plants potentiated at low dosages by what is known in other disciplines as stochastic resonance. (Especially in electronics where acoustic engineers have traditionally sought to minimise noise in the search for the perfect signal, it was found that in certain situations random noise actually improved the output. This noise-to-signal ratio has applications in other informatic settings, notably in low dose pharmacy where traditional remedies from plants have given way to the search for pure molecules free from stochastic effects.)

For my third treatment with a herbalist I had to travel a great distance. The therapeutic approach taken towards me was cognate with the therapeutic approach I had developed over the years towards my own patients and that I had at last taken towards myself this third time. I was prescribed several preparations (none of which I could ever have written for myself) and was gratified to find peace and resolution of a painful condition that had beset me for 30 years. I liked all of the medicines, including the one that contained essential oil of juniper. I had learnt the lessons of dosage and timing.

In explaining my absence from my weekly lesson because of my *crise de foie* all those years ago, I rather gushed about my surprise and delight at the herbal treatment. My Provençal teacher – an octogenarian survivor of the *Résistance* – retorted: 'What else would you expect to do? I am a herbalist too, but I don't make a fuss about it.' In our culture where we cannot take so much for granted, I am very glad that NIMH is making a justifiable fuss about the 150 years of our work with patients and our struggle for recognition in the political arena.

Given how varied and rich are the intercessions between plants and people it is not so easy in herbal medicine to settle on first principles, but the sensuousness of plants will abide: when the arthralgia of old age may cause pain even in the fingers that pick the basil and parsley, the heart at least may be rewarded.

References

Chardenon, L. 1985. *In praise of wild herbs: remedies and recipes from Old Provence*, introduced by Lawrence Durrell. London: Century; originally published in 1973 as *The plant magic man*. Santa Barbara: Capra.

Keen, B. 1941. *Herb gathering*. Brome & Schimmer, Botanical Drug Importers.

Further reading

Barker, J. 1980. *The herbal year book.* London: Eel Pie Publishing.

Barker, J. 2001. *The medicinal flora: field guide to the medicinal plants of Britain and north-western Europe.* West Wickham: Winter Press.

Barker, J. 2007. *History, philosophy and medicine: phytotherapy in context.* West Wickham: Winter Press /UEL.

Barker, J. 2011. *From solstice to equinox and back again: the influence of the midpoint on human health and the use of plants to modify such effects.* Lewes: The Order of Bards Ovates & Druids.

Trunks and leaves

Producing the well rounded herbalist

Christopher Hedley

When each of us started out on our path a seed was sown in our hearts. This seed will grow into a mighty tree. Its roots are in our tradition and in our personal relationship with the earth. Its branches spread far and wide encompassing the many different aspects of our discipline, art and science, poetry and pharmacology. Our leaves draw energy from the air and sun and, at the end of the year, they fall back to the earth to make fresh humus. Or, of course, we could hang onto our leaves; there are many different types of herbalist. Are you an evergreen or a deciduous herbalist? Are you a Pine or a Birch an Oak or an Ash?

Holding everything together is our trunk. Good heartwood at the centre surrounded by a network of fine tubes hastening goodness up and down between the roots and the leaves. I love to look at trees, something that Non Shaw taught me, and see how they grow in relation to each other and to the environment around them. Which way they bend and shape themselves in a slow dance over many years. Trees are very like human beings. They have their feet earthed and their heads reaching to heaven. Of all plants, trees are the easiest for us to relate to, as individuals. Some patients respond very well when asked to find a friendly tree to hang out with and ... I don't necessarily mean demonstrative tree hugging just hanging out is OK.

Plants are our tools, allies and friends. Getting to know them well is the key to herbal practice. Culpeper's dictum, 'English herbs for English bodies', applies as much to the herbalist as to their patients – more so in fact. Getting to know your local herbs, wandering around touching them and talking to them is the sustaining joy in herbal life, whether they are growing in your garden or as 'weeds' from the wild land around. We all have wild land around us even in the centre of our cities. Those small patches growing unexpected treats that make walking down any street with a herbalist such a joyful experience – or maybe just annoying for non-herbalists.

Consider the beauty of a spear thistle rosette early in its first year, watch it accumulate strength and then, over the next year, follow its growth up to those elegant flowers. The base of the flowering heads is tasty food. Thistles are, of course an excellent food for melancholic types, clearing the liver congestion to which they are prone. Reflect on Eeyore eating his thistles – hard work suited to his nature but with the reward of a delicious taste.

Wander down to the park to admire the trees and pick a few sweet pine twigs to make a smudge stick. Five needled pines are best. The sweet smell attracts good spirits – for your own use and for your patients.

The great joy of herbal medicine is the wide variety of methods of application from the most simple, just hanging out with the plants, to complex, multilayered preparations such as alchemical spagyrics. In general the simplest ways, those closest to nature, are the best. Next spring try nibbling the 'bread and cheese' tips from your local hawthorn hedge - without using your hands. That way they taste so much better. Get to know your local plants. That's the key. Even if you finish up using a variety of herbs from around the world in your practice your local plants will strengthen your connection with nature, with the earth itself, and make you a more effective practitioner.

It is possible to make a remedy for just about any complaint from herbs growing within a half hour's walk of any herbalist's home – with the addition of a simple larder from the kitchen. There's a challenge for you next time you go out for a Sunday stroll around the neighbourhood! Grow fresh roots in the rich soil of our herbal traditions. Learn what you can about the history of your favourite herbs, about how our ancestors worked with them. It's a great pleasure to find an old recipe and copy it, expanding your repertoire and turning old insights into new. Here's one for a cordial to help live long taken from Archdale Palmer's recipe book handwritten between 1659 & 1672,

> *'Take a quart of Malaga wine, or any good white Spanish, infuse into it one or two tops of rue, rosemary and sage, and let it simmer*

till about a sixth of a pint has boiled away. Sweeten it with white, crystallised sugar and bottle it. Take 2 or 3 teaspoons at a time - not sipping politely but taking a resolute gulp'

I like that last instruction. How you take a remedy is just as important as how you make it.

Read up the story of a herb – its evolving journey with our own species and create a work of art from it; a poem or a collage, a song or a dance. Have fun! It is too easy to get lost in herbalism as only a serious pursuit. Bring joy to your relationship with plants and you will learn more from them. Take inspiration from the likes of Andy Goldsworthy OBE, a British sculptor, photographer and environmentalist producing land art in Scotland.

Working with the plants, making foods and medicines, is the way of connecting with our herbal ancestors. The first step is harvesting. Each herb requires a different technique. Each technique is slowly, and sometimes painfully, learned. I often think of my ancestors when out picking of how they must draw gentle fun from my clumsy technique. Working with our hands strengthens our hearts and strengthens our herbal trunk.

Working and being with our local plants has the added bonus of keeping us in touch with the seasons. It is far too easy to ignore the flow of the seasons in the hurly burly of modern life, with artificial heating, artificial lighting and artificial distractions all around. But our bodies know. They respond to each seasonal change and being aware of this response is an important part of staying healthy. Live seasonally, eat seasonally, make and take your medicines seasonally and watch how the plants, the earth and your body respond to those changes. Learn what you can about seasonal traditions – the little magical acts our ancestors would do at specific times of the year. At the beginning of the year weave a ball from hawthorn twigs and hang it up for the year coming. The thorns catch onto any negative thoughts and feelings – especially useful if you practise at home. Use this type of simple symbolism in your practice. It is the basis of personal ceremony – a powerful healing tool.

At midsummer collect the traditional herbs and make a wreath to hang over your front door, announcing to the world who you are and what you do. Mugwort is a good start. You can make mugwort pillows for patients with anxiety dreams, full of confused thoughts. Herb pillows are a simple way of bringing a good night's sleep – hops are good for

Choleric (Fire) types whose sleep is disturbed by plans of action rather than by anxiety and lavender is for elders. We all know these things but how often do we actually use them?

And teach what you have learned – in order to learn more! We can all do some sort of teaching; cream making or cookery workshops, herbal walks, talks to local groups. After you have a few years' practice under your belt you may wish to teach at a more advanced level, treating family and friends and even other practitioners. There is a need for this. The academic environment does not suit everyone. It is possible to teach a rigorous course with a lighter, more practical touch and include all the insights you have gleaned from playing with the plants, from developing a solid yet flexible trunk.

Teaching, working with local groups spreads the vital message that we, as a species, must reconnect with nature or we are lost – the earth will move on to its next experiment leaving us behind. Teaching and taking part in local groups and grass roots environmental organisations is the only way to change humanities attitude towards the earth. Whatever happens with Statutory Regulation of herbal practitioners it won't be the answer. As a profession we must put our energy back into developing ourselves as champions of the right way to behave on this earth ... and we should keep an eye on our own practice, thinking carefully about provenance and sustainability. Where do our herbs and tinctures come from? Were they grown and harvested with respect for the earth and for the local community? Ask your professional body to help keep you up to date on environmental issues.

Do all you can to strengthen your trunk and freely give back your leaves to make a new, rich humus for our children and our children's children – for the sake of our ancestors.

References

Uden, G., (ed) *The recipe book, 1659-1672, of Archdale Palmer, Gentl, Lord of the Manor of Wanlip in the county of Leicestershire.* Sandhurst: Sycamore Press.

Further Reading

Hedley, C. and Shaw, N., 2001. *Herbal remedies a practical beginner's guide to making effective remedies in the kitchen.* Bath: Parragon.

Junius, M.M., 1979. *Spagyrics.* Vermont: Healing Arts Press.

Chricton campus and humanities advanced technology and information institute, 2006. *The Andy Goldsworthy digital catalogue.* Available from: http://www.goldsworthy.cc.gla.ac.uk/ (Accessed 28 April 2014)

Green healing
– biophilia, herbal medicine and health

Chanchal Cabrera

There is an instinctive attraction of people to plants – whether a bouquet of flowers, a lovely park, a path through the woods or our own gardens. This is the basis for the practices of both horticulture therapy and of herbal medicine which are, in this sense, merely different aspects of a single plant-based healing experience available to patients. We feel better when we have exposure to plants and we use them for ceremony and celebration. Births and deaths have been marked with flowers for thousands of years, as witness the ancient Persian burial chambers with many seeds and plant remains. Kings and Queens since the ancient Egyptians have been anointed with herbs on ascending to the throne. Even Elizabeth II was anointed with neroli, rose, cinnamon, jasmine, benzoin, musk, civet and ambergris in sesame oil. Plants and people have evolved over the millennia, side by side, sharing air and water and even DNA.

Previously the preserve of arcane mathematicians and perhaps of classically trained artists and architects, the concepts and principles of the Fibonacci sequence, the Golden Ratio and the Golden Angle are now recognised in all living things. From the turn of the DNA helix to the turn of the snail shell, from curl of the tornado to the branching pattern of oak trees, from the spacing of the 'eyes' of the butterfly wing to the spacing of the eyes of a 'pretty' woman, we humans are embedded, hard-wired and pre-coded for a sympathetic and even empathic relationship with the natural world. Quite literally, the shape of the world we inhabit is mirrored in the shapes of our bodies. We are deeply gene-coded for awareness of and attunement to nature that when we are cut off from it or see it being damaged or destroyed, we can literally feel as though a part of us is injured. We have stress responses to environmental depredations that may be physical or mental, from ulcers to anxiety, hypertension to depression.

In 2005 author and educator Richard Louv coined the term 'Nature Deficit Disorder'. He described how the innate, natural and intuitive connections that children feel to the natural world are part of our 'hard-wiring' and that a lack of exposure to nature in modern urban living is leading to a host of behavioural, physical and even spiritual disorders in adults as well as children. This is in keeping with the well accepted principles of biophilia as espoused by Erich Fromm (2000) and elaborated by E.O. Wilson 30 years earlier. Wilson (1984) defines biophilia as 'the urge to affiliate with other forms of life'. His term is still used today, to mean the capacity to feel union or unity, a sense of one-ness, with the natural world; to feel empathy with animals and perhaps plants.

Richard Louv (2011) describes in *The Nature Principle* how, by tapping into the restorative powers of nature, we can: boost mental acuity and creativity; promote health and wellness; build smarter and more sustainable businesses, communities, and economies; and ultimately strengthen human bonds. He suggests, moreover, that this is perhaps the only way we will survive as a species in the future: by learning to truly value and appreciate the intricate balance of nature and to live in harmony with the finite resources of the planet, instead of degrading and depleting them until it threatens our very existence.

We literally produce hormones of happiness and relaxation when we are exposed to nature. We have fewer mental health problems and recover quicker from physical disease when nature is an integral part of the healing process. Children behave better and achieve better learning outcomes when nature is part of the classroom. Prisoners have demonstrated better behaviours when they get to go outside and work in the institution farm.

There is an extensive and ever-growing body of evidence that supports the age-old understanding of Vis medicatrix naturae (the healing power of nature). From the ancient Egyptians on, including Galen, Avicenna and Culpeper, through physiomedicalism and naturopathy, right up to contemporary clinical herbal practice, this primary truism is integral and fundamental to the deep understanding of how herbs work.

An extensive reading list is given for those wishing to understand the science and research behind the healing power of nature. As a medical herbalist since 1987, I was intellectually aware of this and knew how much I personally needed access to nature, to a garden or to the forest for my own well-being. Ironically, I had never connected the dots nor considered the opportunities for clinicians to integrate the concepts of biophilia into clinical practice.

That all changed for me in the summer of 2000 when I was privileged to have an opportunity to experience a personal retreat with an accomplished shamanic practitioner using traditional Amazonian medicine. He soaked the herbs then cooked them up with songs, chants and prayer over several days. After I drank the bitter brew I had a feeling of becoming at one with nature, of becoming a water molecule, ascending through the xylem vessels and being part of photosynthesis. There was no conscious thought or verbal understanding, yet I could feel intensely and absolutely. It was kinaesthetically evident how the annular rings of the xylem vessel spin the plant fluids as they rise, creating the vortex so familiar to biodynamic and homeopathic theory, and at the same time, it exactly and perfectly follows the laws of the Golden Angle. It was way beyond feeling at one with nature; I became one with the natural world and 'I' ceased to be.

In that intensely beautiful moment of perfect unity I was acutely aware that my academic and analytical research and the Master's degree I was pursuing were not sufficient to satisfy an urgent need in me to somehow share this sense of one-ness and of belonging with others. Soon after completing my Masters science degree I took certification in Horticulture Therapy and I have been working with healing gardens ever since. I now believe that one of the unspoken and unofficial but none the less critical roles of the herbalist is to strengthen people's relationship with nature, to assist them to feel connected to the greater whole and to understand their own roles and responsibilities in the natural order. By deepening a patient's appreciation of and concern for nature the patient receives healing on a very deep and profound level, far beyond any chemical constituents or carefully constructed formula. By engaging the biophilia instinct great healing can occur, first on a personal level and from that social and environmental healing can begin to flow.

So on a practical level, what can a clinical herbalist do to foster feelings of biophilia? How can practitioners integrate nature into clinical practice? I suppose that I am lucky in that after many years in a clinic in the city, in a room with a skylight but no window, I now have 7 acres of gardens to grow over 200 medicinal species and enjoy with patients. If you only have a backyard or an allotment garden simply scale back these ideas by choosing the top dozen or two herbs that are easy to grow and that you regularly use and many of them don't require the outdoors at all.

The herbal clinic

When choosing new clinic rooms look for a space that has good natural light for indoor plants, an outdoor space (garden, patio or courtyard), attractive plantings at the entrance

Bring nature indoors – plants (must be kept looking healthy!), floral prints on the wall, fresh flowers on the desk

Have a friendly cat or dog for patients to pet or a beautiful aquarium for restful watching

Ensure that your view is attractive – if there is another building in front of your window then can you have a window box (inside or outside)?

Always offer a cup of herbal tea to encourage patients to 'connect' to nature and not expect 'medicine' to always be in a pill or potion. I always prescribe a tea as part of the herbal protocol to keep people in touch with the plants.

Themed activities to initiate conversations with patients (individually or in groups)

Forest bathing

This is the literal translation of the Japanese term Shin-rin yoku; first used in 1982 and now a generic term for 44 approved nature sites regulated and managed by the Japanese Forest Therapy Executive Committee. The term refers to the practice of mindfulness meditation in forests. It may be accomplished through contemplative walking in the woods, through sitting in silence in the forest, through chanting or singing in the trees. In all cases though, practising being present, in the moment, not caught up in '21st century busy brain', is key to the experience. It is a cell-phone-free experience.

Intentional medicine meditation

The practitioner chooses a plant relevant for the patient to sit with in the garden or the woods, to meditate with and explore inwardly, then discuss and review as appropriate with the practitioner. This may involve expressive arts (drawing or painting the expression of the plant), making a flower remedy or a tea, or using other creative ways of experiencing and learning.

Winter solstice wreath making activity

Keeping the hands busy with a simple creative task allows the mind to wander and the conversation to flow. Making wreaths may engender conversation exploring issues of death, loss and bereavement (metaphors of circles and evergreens and return of the sun). Working with the plant attributions of Dr Edward Bach's flower remedies, holly may initiate a conversation about anger or weaving a willow wreath base may allow a discussion about flexibility and capacity for change. If your patients are able, take them into the woods to harvest the evergreen boughs, mistletoe and holly so they experience forest bathing as well.

Themed herbal planters

Planting up attractive pots for specific conditions, means patients can take home and tend related plants or even harvest some tea that then allows a conversation about the condition. The combinations listed in the table are the planters we are making for our plant nursery this summer. The plants are all easy to grow in a zone 6.5–7.5 and reasonably tolerant of my rather casual gardening style.

Medicinal plant pots

Menopause	motherwort, sage, feverfew, rose & lemon
Headaches	feverfew, betony & skullcap
Skin Care	lavender, marigold, ribwort & violet
Liver	milk thistle, dandelion, celandine & wormwood
Colds and Flu	echinacea, oregano & white horehound,
Lung Tonic	mullein, marshmallow, elecampane & violet
Sleepytime	lemon balm, chamomile, skullcap, valerian & Californian poppy

StressLess	St John's wort, betony, luzea (maral root) & skullcap
Digestease	peppermint, vervain & wormwood
Parasites	wormwood, sage, tansy & fennel

Teatime plant pots

Sweet & Spicy	bee balm, orange spice thyme & lemon balm
Rose Dreams	rose bergamot, rose thyme & rose
Mint Medley	peppermint, spearmint & fruit mint
Chocolate Orange Mint	chocolate mint & orange spice thyme
Wild Weeds Salad Mix	violet, chickweed, sheep sorrel, dandelion, miner's lettuce & purslane
Herb Garden Mix	oregano, thyme, sage, tarragon & fennel
Salad Dressing	rosemary, thyme, savory & chives

Themed herb walks

If planting pots and doing a 'make and take home' workshop is not for you, then perhaps you have some of the plants in your garden or perhaps visit a good botanic garden. If you have access to nature trails, a herb walk can be themed around a condition such as heart health (hawthorn, dandelion, yarrow, linden (lime), daisy and cleavers), or a spring detox theme (burdock, yellow dock, cleavers, wild watercress, violet leaf and dandelion).

Memory garden

This is a special themed planter to be made by someone at end of life and gifted to another with stories around the plants. A memory garden is a container or a bed of flowers or plants that have special significance for the patient. They may be flowers that were favourites of the patient's mother; flowers that were in the patients wedding bouquet; blooms that remind the patient of happier times, etc. It could be made in a garden or pavilion, or can be done in an activity room.

The benefits of planting a memory garden are many:

Physical

Offers pleasant aromas – not disinfectant and medical smells. Toxic cancer treatments often distort the sense of smell and taste and pleasant smelling herbs and flowers can be immensely pleasing to these people

Opportunity for exercise – increased strength and flexibility
Opportunity to be outdoors with increased oxygen and sunlight
Improved dexterity and fine motor control from seeding, weeding, hoeing, etc., and also from later crafting projects

Cognitive
Offers distraction from pain and suffering
Opportunity for a change of scenery – looking at living landscapes instead of walls
Learning opportunity
Feelings of self-worth and self esteem

Emotional
Brings back happy memories
Something to share with others as gifts - ability to give
Opportunity for socialising and conversation
Believing in the future – ordering seeds and waiting for them to sprout then flower

Spiritual
Chance to exercise choice and free will – feeling of being in control
Opportunity to be creative in choosing plants and container
Feeling of hopefulness watching things sprout – a reason to wake up in the morning

Some other ways of bringing in healing with nature aside from ingesting plants in the form of teas or tinctures include: applying plants topically in the form of lotions, salves and foot baths, inhaling plant essential oils in a diffuser, ingesting plants in the form of flower essences, and using plants ritualistically and ceremonially, for example, burning sage or myrrh for purification and frankincense for inviting in fresh energy.

In conclusion

It is now an unassailable fact that people thrive where there are intact and robust natural ecosystems, where they can easily access green space and the natural world, where they engage in less screen time and more outdoor activities. Plants, pets, parks, wilderness and nature are essential requirements for good health of individuals and societies. Doctors Eva Selhub and Alan Logan (2012) called it Vitamin G for 'green' and they prescribe immersion in nature as a daily practice. Medical herbalists are perfectly positioned to be delivering this old – new plant medicine discipline and there are myriad creative ways and means of doing this.

References

Buhner, S., 2002. *Lost language of plants.* Vermont: Chelsea Green.

Buhner, S., 2004. *Secret teachings of plants.* Vermont: Bear and Co.

Lewis, C., 1996. *Green nature human nature.* Champaign, IL: University of Illinois Press.

Lipton, B., 2005. *The biology of belief.* California: Elite Books.

Louv, R., 2005. *Last child in the woods.* North Carolina: Algonquin Books.

Louv, R., 2011. *The nature principle.* North Carolina: Algonquin Books.

Pollan, M., 1991. *Second nature.* New York: Grove Press.

Metzner, R., 1999. *Green psychology.* Vermont: Park Street Press.

Roszak, T., 1992. *The voice of the earth.* Michigan: Phanes Press.

Roszak, T., 1995. *Ecopsychology.* Berkeley, CA: University California Press.

Selhub, E. and Logan, A., 2012. *Your brain on nature.* Toronto: Collins.

Wilson, E.O., 1984. *Biophilia.* Cambridge, MA: Harvard University Press.

Further reading

American Horticultural Association, 2014. Available from http://www.ahta.org [Accessed 20 May 2014].

American Society of Landscape Architects, 2014. Available from http://host.asla.org/groups/tgdpigroup/index.htm [Accessed 20 May 2014].

Cabrera, C., 2002. *Fibromyalgia – a journey toward healing.* New York: Magraw-Hill Contemporary Books.

Canadian Horticultural Therapy Association, 2014. Available from http://www.chta.ca [Accessed 20 May 2014].

Cooper Marcus, C. and Barnes, M., 1999. *Healing gardens: therapeutic benefits and design recommendations.* New York: Wiley Press.

Gerlach-Spriggs, N., Kaufman, R.E. and Warner, S.B., 1998. *Restorative gardens: the healing landscape.* New Haven, CT: Yale University Press.

Kaplan, R. and Kaplan, S., 1989. *The experience of nature: a psychological perspective.* Cambridge University Press.

Kaplan, R., Kaplan, S. and Ryan, R.E., 1998. *With people in mind: design and management of everyday nature*. Washington, DC: Island Press.

Simson, S., ed., 1998. *Horticulture as therapy: principles and practices*. Binghamton, NY: Food Products Press.

Shoemaker, C., ed., 2002. *Interaction by design: bringing people and plants together for health and well-being*. Iowa State Press.

Taylor, E.R., 1994. *The enabling garden: creating barrier-free gardens*. Dallas: Taylor Publishing.

Thrive, 2014. Available from http://www.thrive.org.uk [Accessed 20 May2014].

Trellis, 2014. Available from http://www.trellisscotland.org.uk [Accessed 20 May 2014].

Turner, N.J., 1991. *Common poisonous plants and mushrooms of North America*. Portland, OR: Timber Press.

Wells, S., ed., 1997. *Horticultural therapy and the older adult population*. New York: Haworth Press.

Whitehouse, S., *et al.*, 2001. 'Evaluating a children's hospital garden environment: utilization and consumer satisfaction', *Journal of environmental psychology*, 21, 301- 314.

Sourcing herbs sustainably

Past, present and future?

Anne Stobart

Where do herbal medicines come from? This might seem like a silly question, but when we actually think about it there is a great untold story about how herbal medicines were sourced in the past, where they come from today, and how the future for the supply of medicinal plants may unfold. The National Institute of Medical Herbalists (NIMH) has worked hard to develop and accredit professional training for the practice of herbal medicine, and I consider myself fortunate to have been able to teach herbal medicine at Middlesex University while both in clinical practice and developing my research interests. I have had a particular interest in how herbal supplies have been obtained in the past, and the challenges ahead in ensuring future supplies for the professional practitioner. From the twin standpoints of a historical researcher and organic grower, this article outlines some issues in historical background and some key concerns ahead, with examples of developments with which I have been involved.

It is no surprise that the history of herbal medicine forms a substantial part of the history of medicine, since plants have been the mainstay of health care for households and medical practitioners for millennia. From classical times to the early modern period both self-help household healthcare and professional practice involving apothecaries, physicians and surgeons would have required supplies of correctly identified plants and the right parts – especially difficult to confirm when dried plant material was used. Practitioners, and lay people too, were largely untrained in plant identification and (until the time of Linnaeus) lacking an agreed system for naming plants and so may have consistently recognised only a rather limited number of plants. Concerns about obtaining the right plants of suitable quality extended to the modern general practitioner even in the nineteenth century when the field of pharmacognosy rapidly developed providing both macroscopic and microscopic analytical data for plant recognition and quality (Evans 2009). Within the past 150 years, despite the use of vast quantities of raw materials both home-grown and imported, the commercial synthesis of individual molecules has grown alongside the development of biomedicine, relegating many herbal medicines to a side-line in medical history. Identification and synthesis of plant chemicals early in the nineteenth century, such as morphine and quinine, led to changes in the production of medicines, with an increasing shift from whole-plant extracts to pure single-constituent drugs. For example, salicin in willow bark was first identified in the early nineteenth century; synthetically made acetylsalicylic acid, with a trade name of aspirin, was first commercially produced in Germany in 1874 (Arteca 1996). In the UK, the previously-named Wholesale Drug Trade Association became the Association of the British Pharmaceutical Industry in 1961, a reflection of the changes in the nature of the business which included much research effort to identify new medicines (Corley 1999/2000, Newman and Cragg 2007, Richmond *et al.* 2003).

Many people probably assume that, in the past, herbs were widely available in the field and hedgerow, or could be grown in the garden, and so fail to consider questions about bulk supplies of herbs in commerce whether harvested in the UK or imported. Pharmaceutical businesses, such as Boots, developed from medical botany businesses which responded to a demand for remedies for self-medication (Holloway 1991), but there was heavy reliance on imports and disruptions in supplies could affect arrangements significantly (Griggs 1981). My very first piece of historical investigation concerned how local people in a Wiltshire town were encouraged by their schoolteacher to gather herb supplies because of a problem with imports between the First and Second World Wars (Stobart 1998). It was striking that the gatherers made little use of the herbs themselves, but preferred to nip down to the local chemist for pharmaceutically prepared remedies. But there are indications that a range of medicinal plants were grown commercially in the UK not so long ago, and some in significant quantities – for example, liquorice – although there are few details of past practices in cultivation and harvesting (Grieve 1980).

When I started looking for source material for this article, I was reminded just how little reliable historical information on herbal supplies is readily accessible. Indeed, research into the history of herbal medicine as a whole has been fragmented, with much material constantly repeated without checking, and there are many areas crying out for further scholarly investigation and links (Stobart and Francia 2014). Some beginnings have been made through a small group of herbal practitioners, the Herbal History Research Network which is committed to encouraging scholarly research. With support from a variety of organisations, including Middlesex University, the NIMH Education Fund, and the Wellcome Trust, we have been bringing active researchers together in seminars since 2010, and in this year of celebration we have planned a further event for researchers with an interest in the history of plant identification and illustration. As the links grow between museum curators, archivists and herbarium managers, social and medical historians, archaeologists, ethnobotanists and others, we hope to recover more detail of the past through studies of people, plants and practices. One major step forward has been the publication of an edited collection of some of the herbal history seminar papers, which represents a welcome collaboration between researchers in different disciplines (Francia and Stobart 2014).

Looking ahead, environmental changes due to global warming and new patterns of land use are impacting on biodiversity and, potentially, affecting supplies of herbal medicines. The World Health Organisation is widely quoted as stating that plant medicines still serve the majority of the world population (although most countries now have significant elements of biomedicine alongside traditional systems) and has sought to provide guidance to regulate the quality of harvested materials (World Health Organisation 2003). Meanwhile demand for herbal medicines has also been increasing in the industrialised nations. There are two key areas that need to be considered in thinking ahead. Firstly, the issue of sustainability – this requires recognition of sustainably managed sources through mechanisms like regulatory standards for wild harvests, and organic accreditation for cultivated supplies. However, organic accreditation possibilities are still limited for non-timber forest products (NTFPs). Secondly, there is an issue about the extent of self-sufficiency – the ability to cultivate and harvest our own supplies in the UK, in a cost-effective way, which includes developing the infrastructure to support sufficient supply and demand. This involves both recovering details of past practices and developing new knowledge through pilot studies and experimentation in how to be more self-sufficient.

Sustainability of herbal supplies is a worry. In a comprehensive article for the Herb Society, Sue Minter identified the top 300 medicinal plants and concerns about their supply in the longer term (2009). She noted that the UK is a significant importer, at eleventh on the world list of herbal importers. Raw plant materials are still shipped all over the world and trade now involves billions of Euros both in imports and exports (European Federation of Pharmaceutical Industries and Associations 2013) through a relatively small number of key market centres such as Hamburg in Germany. A breakdown of statistical detail on this world trade is not readily available as the categories of medicinal natural products overlap with categories for products used in perfumery and cosmetics, and other categories relating to essential oils, gums and resins. There is a specific category for some 'medicinal plants' (coded 1211) which records a world level of exports for 2012 of nearly US$ 2.7 billion of which almost one-third is exported from China (International Trade Centre 2014). This is likely an underestimate of the overall trade, most of which is wild-harvested. Concerns about sustainability in herbal supplies from less developed countries have underpinned calls for regulation (Vines and Behrens 2004). Today, increased levels of medicinal plant regulation to protect the wild harvest should benefit herbal practitioners and patients in terms of certifying the quality of supplies, and protect the rights of indigenous peoples to make a sustainable income. The new Fairwild standards provide considerable protection for both plants and people's livelihoods (Kathe 2011) – but there is quite a hurdle in ensuring education for growers and suppliers to understand and use these standards, and for patients and consumers to appreciate the need to properly protect the sources (which comes at a cost). Imports and exports of raw plant materials for cosmetic and health uses are largely managed for and by multinational corporations, and relatively few small-scale businesses are continuing to provide supplies for the clinical herbal practitioner. These businesses have valiantly worked to improve the quality of herbal supplies, to respond to regulatory changes and to continue to serve herbal practitioners. Here we can see that herbal practitioners and herbal growers and manufacturers have interests in common, and the importance of continuing with ongoing links through NIMH.

Self-sufficiency could be further developed – whether drawing on past practices, learning from the example of others, or experimenting to establish what we can cultivate and harvest successfully in the UK. Not so long ago, herbal practitioners like myself would have been looking at our dispensary shelves at bottles with labels showing their distant sources – for example hawthorn (*Crataegus oxyacantha*) berry tincture from eastern Europe – and wondering why we needed to import something which grows so readily in the UK? Many herbal practitioners already grow or harvest some herb supplies, although the focus tends to be garden or hedgerow plants on an individual scale. So far, one survey to look at the viability of UK-based commercial developments in plants has suggested that there are few possibilities worth considering (Sanderson and Prendergast 2002): though perhaps this view arose because this survey considered mainly coppice and craft trades rather than potential medicinal and health markets. There has been far more encouragement in the USA for local growers and landowners to gain spinoffs from their lands (Vance and Thomas 1997). In this connection, US organisations like United Plant Savers (UPS) have sought to establish a network of botanical sanctuaries which highlight the diversity of medicinal plants and the potential for sustainable cultivation. For example ginseng and goldenseal, both woodland plants highly threatened by illegal but profitable wild harvesting, present opportunities for cultivation and harvest producing high-quality dried roots. In 2010, I was fortunate to visit the UPS Ohio-based botanical sanctuary and see this work at first hand, and to experience a real sense of expanding possibilities. During my visit I saw other inspiring developments such as the nearby Community Kitchen at Athens, Ohio. This was not just an extended bakery but a location where small businesses could access commercial-scale dryers, freezers, processing and storage facilities for realistic rental rates. Such facilities have enabled a number of small businesses, including one supplying a range of herbal medicinal teas, to establish and grow with success (Appalachian Center for Economic Networks 2014).

History may not provide all the answers about practices of cultivation and harvest of medicinal plants – for example, I have found no records about coppicing trees and shrubs for medicinal use in the UK – so we have to experiment to find out what works in practical ways. I am a co-founder of a project at Holt Wood in North Devon which represents a very personal commitment to gaining knowledge and skills in sustainable cultivation of medicinal trees and shrubs. Starting with a private purchase of land in 2005, we cleared an area of two acres of Sitka Spruce and replanted with native and introduced trees and shrubs to provide medicinal supplies alongside timber, fuel and food crops. Using permaculture design principles, we created wide rides and many woodland 'edges' in which light-demanding shrubs and wildflowers can flourish. The project has since been recognised by the Permaculture Association as one of their innovative LAND network of demonstration projects helping to educate others about possibilities. We have been experimenting with coppicing and pollarding of cramp bark (*Viburnum opulus* L.) and willow (*Salix alba* L. and *Salix daphnoides* Vill.) to find more efficient ways of harvesting and processing bark. Other introduced shrubs which have grown well include prickly ash bark (*Zanthoxylum americanum* Mil.) and witch hazel (*Hamamelis virginiana* L.). Through open days and courses, as well as blogs and articles, we have sought to enthuse others in the possibilities of producing medicinal supplies alongside other woodland products. There is already considerable interest in this project, and many others are active amongst the herbal community in developing gardens, hedgerow harvesting and more (eg, Bruton-Seal and Seal 2008). However, we could be thinking about the bigger picture and whether we can work towards changing the reliance on mass consumption of natural products in the high street which may have been shipped hundreds or thousands of miles. One of our achievements is a first in Devon, the cultivation and production of distilled witch hazel. Much further development is needed to enable more substantial marketing possibilities – including cooperative ventures between growers, accreditation for medicinal tree and shrub products, processing facilities, links with manufacturers, etc.

In conclusion, the last 25 years have been exciting for me in pressing forward with developments in herbal history research and in cultivating medicinal trees and shrubs. For my part, I think this has been considerably helped by the unity and commitment of herbal colleagues. Understanding our tradition in a scholarly way and ensuring the future of herbal medicine supplies are both vital to our profession and, with others in both the academic and business world, I hope we can work towards increasing sustainability and self-sufficiency to match the high standards of NIMH practitioners.

References

Appalachian Center for Economic Networks (ACEnet), 2014. *ACEnet facilities* [online]. Available from: http://www.acenetworks.org/facilities/ [Accessed 22 March 2014].

Arteca, R. N., 1996. *Plant growth substances: principles and applications*. New York: Chapman and Hall.

Bruton-Seal, J., and Seal, M., 2008. *Hedgerow medicine: harvest and make your own herbal remedies*. Ludlow: Merlin Unwin Books.

Corley, T.A.B., 1999/2000. *The British pharmaceutical industry since 1851*. University of Reading.

European Federation of Pharmaceutical Industries and Associations, 2013. *The pharmaceutical industry in figures. Key data – 2013*. Brussels: the European Federation of Pharmaceutical Industries and Associations.

Evans, W.C., 2009. *Trease and Evans' pharmacognosy*. 16th ed. Edinburgh: Elsevier.

Francia, S., and Stobart, A., Eds. 2014. *Critical approaches to the history of Western herbal medicine: from classical antiquity to the early modern period*. London: Bloomsbury.

Grieve, M., 1980. *A modern herbal: the medicinal, culinary, cosmetic and economic properties, cultivation and folklore of herbs, grasses, fungi, shrubs and trees with all their modern scientific uses*. London: Penguin.

Griggs, B., 1981. *Green pharmacy: the history and evolution of Western herbal medicine*. Rochester, Vermont: Healing Arts Press.

Holloway, S.W.F., 1991. *Royal Pharmaceutical Society of Great Britain, 1841-1991: a political and social history*. London: The Pharmaceutical Press.

International Trade Centre, 2014. Trade map. International trade statistics. Product: 1211 medicinal plants [online]. Available from: http://www.trademap.org/tradestat/Country_-SelProduct_TS.aspx [Accessed 6 April 2014].

Kathe, W., 2011. The new FairWild standard – a tool to ensure sustainable wild-collection of plants. *Medicinal plant conservation*, 14, 14–17.

Minter, S., 2009. '*High street herbals: The top 300 over-the-counter herbal medicinals available in the UK: the conservation concerns*' [online].
Available from: http://www.herbsociety.org.uk/members/downloads/300-herbs-minter.pdf [Accessed 31 March 2014].

Newman, D., and Cragg, G., 2007. Natural products as sources of new drugs over the last 25 years. *Journal of natural products*, 70, 461–477.

Richmond, L., Stevenson, J., and Turton, A., 2003. *The pharmaceutical industry: a guide to historical records*. Aldershot: Ashgate.

Sanderson, H., and Prendergast, H.D.V., 2002. *Commercial uses of wild and traditionally managed plants in England and Scotland.* Kew: Centre for Economic Botany, Royal Botanic Gardens.

Stobart, A., and Francia, S., 2014. Conclusion: the history of herbal medicine as a developing field. In: Francia, S., and Stobart, A. Eds. *Critical approaches to the history of Western herbal medicine: from classical antiquity to the early modern period.* London: Bloomsbury, 289–298.

Stobart, A., 1998. Herb collecting in England between the world wars. *European journal of herbal medicine*, 4, (2), 35–38.

Vance, N.C., and Thomas, J., Eds., 1997. *Special forest products: biodiversity meets the marketplace.* Washington DC: US Department of Agriculture, Forest Service.

Vines, G., and Behrens, J., 2004. *Herbal harvests with a future: towards sustainable sources for medicinal plants.* Salisbury: Plantlife International.

World Health Organization, 2003. *WHO guidelines on good agricultural and collection practices (GACP) for medicinal plants.* Geneva: World Health Organization.

Further Reading

Stobart, A., 2013. '"Lett her refrain from all hott spices": medicinal recipes and advice in the treatment of the King's Evil in seventeenth-century south-west England'. *In*: DiMeo, M., and Pennell, S. Eds. *Reading and writing recipe books, 1600–1800.* Manchester University Press, 203–224.

Francia, S., and Stobart, A., eds., 2014. *Critical approaches to the history of Western herbal medicine.* London: Bloomsbury.

Herbal Therapeutics

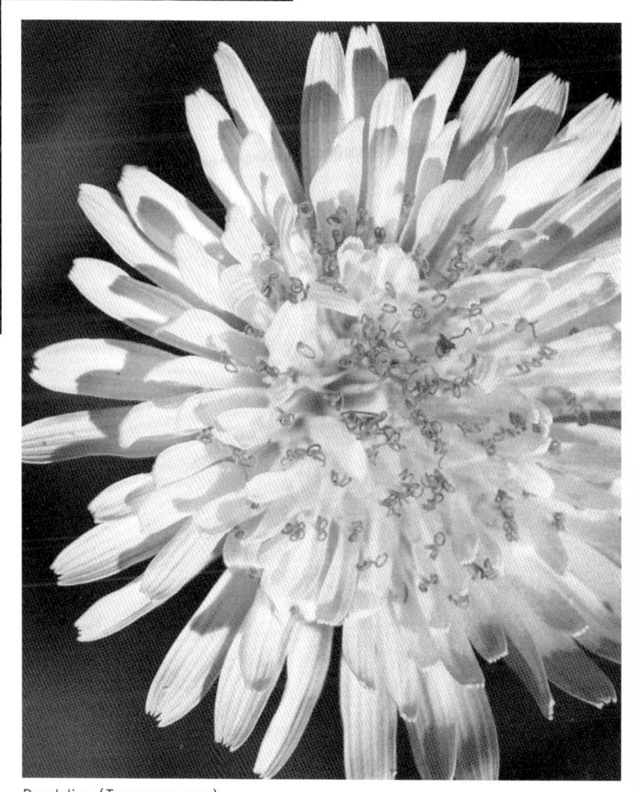

Dandelion (*Taraxacum* spp.)

Managing the menace of antimicrobial resistance with herbal medicine

Michael McIntyre

On 30 April 2014 the World Health Organisation (WHO) published its first global report on antimicrobial resistance (AMR), revealing that AMR was now a serious major worldwide threat to public health occurring in every region of the world, potentially affecting anyone, of any age, in any country. Dr Keiji Fukuda, WHO's Assistant Director-General for Health Security, warned that, if measures were not taken immediately to counter AMR, 'the implications will be devastating... Without urgent, coordinated action by many stakeholders, the world is headed for a post-antibiotic era, in which common infections and minor injuries which have been treatable for decades can once again kill' (WHO 2014). This stark warning echoed a similar apocalyptic alert issued by the Chief Medical Officer for England, Professor Dame Sally Davies, who declared that the danger posed by growing resistance to antibiotics was 'a ticking time bomb' that should be ranked along with terrorism on a list of threats to the nation (Walsh 2013).

It is a striking omission that in its list of recommendations to counter AMR, WHO made no mention of using traditional herbal medicines. Yet herbal medicine is likely to have a significant role to play in combating the growing threat of AMR and cannot be marginalised any longer. The term 'orphan drug' has entered the lexicon describing any drug whose sales would fail to generate sufficient returns for the pharmaceutical industry to justify the investment needed for its development (see EMA definition; EMA 2014). Yet in herbal medicine, we encounter another phenomenon – an entire 'orphan therapy' – since investment available

The 2014 WHO report highlights seven bacteria responsible for common, serious diseases becoming resistant to treatment (WHO 2014)	
Escherichia coli	causing bloodstream infections (sepsis), urinary tract infections, food-borne infections
Klebsiella pneumoniae	pneumonia and other respiratory infections, bloodstream infections (sepsis), urinary tract infections, wound infections
Methicillin-resistant *Staphylococcus aureus* (MRSA)	skin infections, wound infections, bloodstream infections (sepsis), septic arthritis
Streptococcus pneumoniae	pneumonia, meningitis, sinusitis and otitis media, cellulitis, brain abscess
Nontyphoidal *Salmonella*	diarrhoea
Shigella species	diarrhoea and dysentery
Neisseria gonorrhoeae	gonorrhoea

for funding the testing and development of drugs is dependent on providing dividends for shareholders who can expect no return on herbal medicines which, occurring naturally, cannot be patented. The legal and financial structures of the UK and EU appear institutionally and structurally biased against herbal medicine and its practice; the funding that underpins research into conventional pharmaceuticals is not available for the development of herbal medicine or its practice.

Another bias against herbal medicine arises from medicine's focus on killing off infective organisms, be they bacteria, fungi or viruses, largely ignoring the terrain in which the infection takes root. Herbal medicines do not have the potency of powerful antibiotics and so have been mostly ignored as a resource to treat infections. Medicine developed this way because it adopted the philosophical perspectives on health and disease of Robert Koch (1843–1910) who declared bacteria to be 'the smallest but most dangerous enemies of mankind' (Gradmann 2000) and disregarded the views of Max Josef von Pettenkofer (1818–

1901) who famously drank a cholera cocktail cultured from a dead patient without falling ill to demonstrate that the cholera germ infects those weakened with a poor diet or constitution. Instead, medicine was entirely driven by the 'germ theory' of disease promulgated by Louis Pasteur (1822–1885) and modern antibiotics can be said to be a vindication of this approach. However, in just a few decades, we have squandered the effectiveness of antibiotics by inappropriate overuse in humans and animals. Medical research has been focused on the most potent way to kill germs with few resources devoted to exploring how to raise the effectiveness of the immune system, but now AMR threatens our way of life, demanding that society adopts new perspectives and strategies to manage infection.

Responding to this threat calls for the adoption of sustainable strategies that will avoid the development of antimicrobial resistance to medicines we use. The famous Daoist concept '*wei wu wei: action without action*' is a practical strategy worthy of exploration. Indeed, it is an important feature of herbal medicine; plant medicines can be utilised to revitalise the sick and vulnerable and so indirectly but effectively raise their resistance to infection. The famous Chinese medical text, *Shen Nong Ben Cao Jing* (Divine Farmer's Materia Medica) written between 300 BCE and 200 CE divided herbal medicines into four categories, the first of which, designated as 'ruler herbs' (*Chen*), are said to have no medicinal effectiveness, ie not directly combating disease but instead strengthening the vitality (*Qi*) of the individual. The Divine Farmer's Materia Medica advised that these 'ruler' herbs should be taken over a long period of time to supplement the body's innate powers of restoration and recuperation, thereby prolonging life. The lower classes of medicines, on the other hand, called assistants (*Zuo*) and aides (*Shi*) displayed marked medicinal effectiveness, ie combating specific diseases, and consequently the ancient materia medica advised they should only be used for a short time for fear of provoking disruption to the system (Unschuld 1986). 2000 years later, these 'ruler' herbs are the tonics herbalists regularly use in their practices, such as panax (*Panax ginseng* C. A. Mey.), astragalus (*Astragalus membranaceus* (Fisch.) Bunge) and the reishi mushroom (*Ganoderma lucidum*), all of which have demonstrable immune-supporting properties helping to ward off infections – *wei wu wei* in practice (Kim *et al.* 2014a, Kim *et al.* 2014b). Astragalus has antiviral properties too; in this case the polysaccharides in the root are believed to be largely responsible for its wide range of actions (Jin *et al.* 2014).

While herbal medicines may not be as powerful as modern antibiotics, they do have effective antibacterial properties. In general, medicinal plants are more effective against gram-positive than gram-negative bacteria (Shan *et al.* 2007). The main antibacterial constituents in botanical medicines are phenols (flavonoids being the largest group): tellingly plants appear to synthesize phenolic compounds in response to pathogen and insect attack, UV radiation and wounding (Korkina 2007). Phenols from spices are active against *Bacillus cereus*, *Listeria monocytogenes*, *Staphylococcus aureus*, *Escherichia coli* and *Salmonella anatum* (Shan *et al.* 2007). However, the non-phenolic constituents of essential oils from oregano, clove, cinnamon, garlic, coriander, rosemary and sage have proved effective against both gram-positive and gram-negative bacteria (Shan *et al.* 2007).

Herbal medicines have been used as antimicrobials for thousands of years, yet they remain effective and this suggests that bacteria, fungi and viruses have a reduced ability to adapt to a plant-derived antimicrobial regime. This is likely to be due to the synergistic effect of the orchestra of chemicals contained by medicinal plants that prevents bacteria, fungi and viruses from developing immunity to their constituents as multi-targeting by the chemical combinations increases efficacy and reduces resistance. The antimicrobial action of each individual herbal medicine is further enhanced by the use of herb combinations routinely employed in all herbal traditions. Synergy occurs at both a pharmacodynamic (what the drug does to the body) and pharmacokinetic (what the body does to the drug) level (Gibbs 2013, Teucher *et al.* 2004) and a number of papers have been published investigating potential benefits conferred by the synergism of phytoconstituents (Bishayee *et al.* 2012, Ricciardiello *et al.* 2011, Fiebich *et al.* 2011, Gertsch 2011, Yang *et al.* 2014).

Synergism can be seen at work where plant medicines are combined with conventional antibiotics to combat AMR and there is a burgeoning body of literature exploring the therapeutic possibilities of this strategy. Most research to find agents to support antibiotics now found ineffective against common bacteria has been lab-based rather than on human populations. A recent review provided evidence of 34 different herbs containing constituents known to inhibit the bacterial efflux pumps (for explanation of this mechanism see below) and thereby potentially reactivate antibiotics to which bacteria have developed immunity (Kourtesi *et al.* 2013). For example, *E. coli* is currently demonstrating resistance to several antibiotics but, combined with extracts of *Sophora alopecuroides* L., isolates of the bacteria were found to be susceptible to ciprofloxacin (Zhou *et al.* 2012). Comparable results were also found employing *Scutellaria baicalensis* Georgi against *S. aureus* to restore the antibacterial actions of ciprofloxacin via similar mechanisms of efflux pump inhibition (Chan *et al.* 2011a).

Another major concern is the drug-resistant bacterium, methicillin-resistant *S. aureus* (MRSA). Exposure to berberine, a compound found in many medicinal plants (eg, *Berberis vulgaris* L., *Coptis chinensis* Franch. and *Phellodendron amurense* Rupr.) together with antibiotics such as levofloxacin and azithromycin (which had recently been proved ineffective against MRSA), resulted in the reactivation of the efficacy of the antibiotic drugs (Zuo *et al.* 2012). Synergistic effects between silibinin (extracted from *Silybum marianum* L. Gaertn.) and antibiotics have also shown potential to inhibit MRSA (Kang *et al.* 2011). Herb-drug combinations are proving effective against other drug-resistant bacteria. Synergistic interaction between epigallocatechin gallate (EGCg) from green tea and antimycotics such as amphotericin B and fluconazole has been reported against *Candida albicans* (Hemaiswarya *et al.* 2008), while *Nigella sativa* L. and omeprazole compared favourably to triple therapy in eradication of *Helicobacter pylori* in 88 patients with dyspepsia and a positive *H. pylori* test (Salem *et al.* 2010).

The ability of herbs to combat antibacterial resistance is achieved in four main ways: firstly by means of a combined phytochemical and antibiotic attack on the bacterial cell wall. For example, carvacrol is a phenol in oregano and thyme that acts as a so-called 'membrane stabiliser', breaching the defensive cell membrane of bacteria and enabling antibiotics to penetrate and destroy gram-negative bacteria (Wagner and Ulrich-Merzenich 2009, Gill and Holley 2006). This mechanism is also responsible for the antifungal properties of carvacrol and thymol against fluconazole-resistant *Candida* isolates (Ahmad *et al.* 2011).

Secondly, antibiotic resistance can be overcome by inhibition of enzymes that are generated by bacteria for the deactivation of antibiotics – EGCg from green tea is active here (Wagner and Ulrich-Merzenich 2009). Thirdly by disabling an efflux pumping system (as mentioned above) developed by bacteria in order to prevent potentially destructive compounds such as antibiotics from penetrating into the bacteria, or to expel the antibiotics out of the bacteria cell once they have invaded it (Wagner and Ulrich-Merzenich 2009). Thyme contains baicalein, which is also present in the *Scutellaria* species (Lamiaceae family), and baicalein has shown significant ability to reverse MRSA resistance to the antibiotic ciprofloxacin by inhibiting the bacteria's defensive efflux pump (Chan *et al.* 2011a).

Bacteria have evolved extraordinary defence systems that would not be out of place in a Star Wars movie and the strategy employed by bacteria to defend against attack by the host's immune system or antibiotic drugs, termed 'quorum sensing' (QS), is a case in point. QS is bacterial signalling that enables bacteria to coordinate defence against compounds toxic to the bacteria. Bacteria use QS to coordinate their activities, such as biofilm formation, virulence, and antibiotic resistance, based on the local density of the bacterial population. Biofilm formation is the production of a protective matrix around the bacterial colony made of polymers – substances composed of molecules with repeating structural units that are connected by chemical bonds. This forms a semi-fluid, glue-like substance that anchors bacteria to animal tissue or any other surface providing a physical barrier that inhibits any attack on the bacteria. As well as occurring within a single bacterial species, QS can be used by diverse species of bacteria to form a mutual defensive biofilm. Unfortunately, medical devices provide the perfect breeding ground for the development of opportunistic bacterial infections and biofilm formation, presenting a secure niche for the proliferation of resistant bacteria (Reid 1999). The fourth method by which herbs can combat antibacterial resistance involves blocking the QS system to help to reduce the virulence of bacteria and prevent the formation of biofilms. Garlic, rosemary, thyme, oregano, sage, basil, cloves cranberry and pomegranate, amongst others, have all been shown to inhibit QS (Nagy 2010).

Of course, herbal medicines can help to resolve the problem of antibiotic resistance more directly. Doctors faced with relatively minor, often self-limiting but common infections, for example, pharyngitis, laryngitis and tonsillitis, or mild urinary tract infections (UTIs) have little to offer except advice on how to manage the condition or otherwise prescribe an antibiotic that may not be appropriate. Herbal medicines fill this therapeutic gap, providing effective treatment that reduces antibiotic prescribing and does not contribute to microbial resistance. For example, a number of herbal medicines are traditionally used to treat sore throat such as sage (*Salvia officinalis* L.) (Hubbert *et al.* 2006, Schapowal *et al.* 2009), dyers woad (*Isatis tinctoria* L.) (Roxas and Jurenka 2007), echinacea (*Echinacea purpurea* L. Moench or *Echinacea angustifolia* DC.) (Sharma *et al.* 2010) and burdock (*Arctium lappa* L.) (Chan *et al.* 2011b, Watkins *et al.* 2012). Herbal medicine can also help to ease UTIs, employing remedies such as bearberry (*Arctostaphylos uva ursi* (L.) Spreng.) (Yarnell 2002, EMA 2012, Larsson *et al.* 1993) and cornsilk (*Zea mays* L.) (Rafsanjany *et al.* 2013), and African geranium (*Pelargonium sidoides* DC.) is effective for treating respiratory infections (Ulbricht *et al.* 2010).

Other common minor infections may also be successfully treated with herbal medicines sparing use of more potent antibiotics. This is a rich territory worth exploring as a cost-efficient and effective way of combating microbial resistance to conventional antimicrobials.

References

Ahmad, A., *et al.*, 2011. Fungicidal activity of thymol and carvacrol by disrupting ergosterol biosynthesis and membrane integrity against *Candida. European journal of clinical microbiology and infectious disease* 30 (1), 41–50.

Bishayee, A., *et al.*, 2012. Dietary phytochemicals in the chemoprevention and treatment of hepatocellular carcinoma: *in vivo* evidence, molecular targets, and clinical relevance. *Current cancer drug targets.* 12 (9), 1191–232.

Chan, B.C., *et al.*, 2011a. Synergistic effects of baicalein with ciprofloxacin against NorA over-expressed methicillin-resistant *Staphylococcus aureus* (MRSA) and inhibition of MRSA pyruvate kinase. *Journal of ethnopharmacology.* 137 (1), 767–73.

Chan, Y.S., *et al.*, 2011b. A review of the pharmacological effects of *Arctium lappa* (burdock). *Inflammopharmacology.* 19 (5), 245–54.

EMA, 2012. Assessment report on *Arctostaphylos uva-ursi* (L.) Spreng., folium, 24 January 2012. *EMA/HMPC/573462/2009 Rev.1* (HMPC).

EMA, 2014. *Orphan Designation.* European Medicines Agency. Available from: http://www.ema.europa.eu/ema/index.jsp?curl=pages/regulation/general/general_content_000029.jsp&. [Accessed 5 May 2014].

Fiebich, B.L., *et al.*, 2011. Pharmacological studies in an herbal drug combination of St. John's wort (*Hypericum perforatum*) and passion flower (*Passiflora incarnata*): *in vitro* and in vivo evidence of synergy between *Hypericum* and *Passiflora* in antidepressant pharmacological models. *Fitoterapia.* 82 (3), 474–80.

Gertsch, J., 2011. Botanical drugs, synergy, and network pharmacology: forth and back to intelligent mixtures. *Planta medica.* 77 (11), 1086–98.

Gibbs, R., 2013. Evaluating the biological actions of Chinese medicinal herbs. *Register of*

Chinese herbal medicine journal. 10, 31–38.

Gill, A.O., and Holley, R.A., 2006. Disruption of *Escherichia coli, Listeria monocytogenes* and *Lactobacillus sakei* cellular membranes by plant oil aromatics. *International journal of food microbiology* 2006 108 (1), 1–9.

Gradmann, C., 2000. Invisible enemies: Bacteriology and the language of politics in imperial Germany. *Science in context.* 13 (1), 9–30.

Hayek, S.A., Gyawali, R., and Ibrahim, S.A., 2013. *Antimicrobial natural products, microbial pathogens and strategies for combating them: science, technology and education* (A. Méndez-Vilas, Ed.). Formatex Research Center.

Hemaiswarya, S., Kruthiventi, A.K., and Doble, M., 2008. Synergism between natural products and antibiotics against infectious diseases. *Phytomedicine.* 15 (8), 639–52.

Hubbert, M., *et al.*, 2006. Efficacy and tolerability of a spray with *Salvia officinalis* in the treatment of acute pharyngitis – a randomised, double-blind, placebo-controlled study with adaptive design and interim analysis. *European journal of medical research.* 11 (1), 20–6.

Jin, M., *et al.*, 2014. Structural features and biological activities of the polysaccharides from *Astragalus membranaceus. International journal of biological macromolecules.* 64, 257–66.

Kang, H.K., Kim, H.Y., and Cha, J.D., 2011. Synergistic effects between silibinin and antibiotics on methicillin-resistant *Staphylococcus aureus* isolated from clinical specimens. *Biotechnology journal.* 6 (11), 1397–408.

Kim, B.H., *et al.*, 2014a. Anti-inflammatory activity of compounds isolated from *Astragalus sinicus L.* in cytokine-induced keratinocytes and skin. *Experimental and molecular medicine.* 21, 46.

Kim, H., *et al.*, 2014b. Immunological activity of ginseng is enhanced by solid-state culture with *Ganoderma lucidum* mycelium. *Journal of medicinal food.* 17 (1), 150–60.

Korkina, L.G., 2007. Phenylpropanoids as naturally occurring antioxidants: From plant defense to human health. *Cellular and molecular biology* 53 (1), 15–25.

Kourtesi, C., *et al.*, 2013. Drug discovery and the challenge of clinical implementation. *Open microbiology journal.* 7 (S:1M3) 34–52.

Larsson, B., Jonasson, A., and Fianu, S., 1993. Prophylactic effect of UVA-E in women with recurrent cystitis: A preliminary report. *Current therapeutic research.* 53 (4), 441–3.

Nagy, M.M., 2010. *Quorum sensing inhibitory activities of various folk-medicinal plants and the thyme-tetracycline effect.* Biology Dissertations. 90. Georgia State University.

Rafsanjany, N., *et al.*, 2013. Antiadhesion as a functional concept for protection against uropathogenic *Escherichia coli: in vitro* studies with traditionally used plants with antiadhesive activity against uropathognic *Escherichia coli. Journal of ethnopharmacology.* 145 (2), 591–7.

Reid, G. 1999. Biofilms in infectious disease and on medical devices. *International journal of antimicrobial agents.* 11, 223-226.

Ricciardiello, L., Bazzoli, F., and Fogliano, V., 2011. Phytochemicals and colorectal cancer prevention – myth or reality? *Nature reviews gastroenterology hepatology.* 8 (10), 592–6.

Roxas, M., Jurenka, J., 2007. Colds and influenza – a review of diagnosis and conventional, botanical and nutritional considerations. *Alternative medicine review.* 12(1), 25–48.

Salem, E.M., *et al.*, 2010. Comparative study of *Nigella sativa* and triple therapy in eradication of *Helicobacter pylori* in patients with non-ulcer dyspepsia. *Saudi journal of gastroenterology.* 16 (3), 207–14.

Schapowal, A., *et al.*, 2009. Echinacea/sage or chlorhexidine/lidocaine for treating acute sore throats: a randomized double-blind trial. *European journal of medical research.* 14 (9), 406–12.

Shan, B., *et al.*, 2007. The *in vitro* antibacterial activity of dietary spice and medicinal herb extracts. *International journal of food microbiology.* 117, 112.

Sharma, S.M., *et al.*, 2010. Bactericidal and anti-inflammatory properties of a standardized echinacea extract (Echinaforce): Dual actions against respiratory bacteria. *Phytomedicine.* 2010 17 (8–9), 563–8.

Teucher, B., Olivares, M., and Cori, H., 2004. Enhancers of iron absorption: ascorbic acid and other organic acids. *International journal for vitamin and nutrition research.* 74, 403–419.

Ulbricht, C., *et al.*, 2010. An evidence-based systematic review of umckaloabo (*Pelargonium sidoides*) by the Natural Standard Research Collaboration. *Journal of dietary supplements.* 7 (3), 283–302.

Unschuld, P., 1986. *Medicine in China – a history of pharmaceutics.* Oakland: University of California Press.

Wagner, H., and Ulrich-Merzenich, G., 2009. Synergy research: approaching a new generation of phytopharmaceuticals. *Phytomedicine.* 16 (2–3), 97–110. Review part 1.

Walsh, F., 2013. *Antibiotics resistance 'as big a risk as terrorism' – medical chief* [online]. BBC News, 11 March 2013. Available from: http://www.bbc.co.uk/news/health-21737844. [Accessed 26 May 2014].

Watkins, F., *et al.*, 2012. Antimicrobial assays of three native British plants used in Anglo-Saxon medicine for wound healing formulations in 10th century England. *Journal of ethnopharmacology.* 144 (2), 408–15.

World Health Organisation, 2014. *WHO's first global report on antibiotic resistance reveals serious, worldwide threat to public health.* Available from: http://www.who.int/mediacentre/news/releases/2014/amr-report/en/. [Accessed 5 May 2014].

Yang, Y., *et al.*, 2014. Synergy effects of herb extracts: pharmacokinetics and pharmacodynamic basis. *Fitoterapia.* 92, 133–47.

Yarnell, E., 2002. Botanical medicines for the urinary tract. *World journal of urology.* 20 (5), 285–93.

Zhou, X., *et al.*, 2012. Total alkaloids of *Sophorea alopecuroides*-induced down-regulation of AcrAB-TolC efflux pump reverses susceptibility to ciprofloxacin in clinical multidrug resistant *Escherichia coli* isolates. *Phytotherapy research.* 26 (11), 1637–43.

Zuo, G.Y., *et al.*, 2012. Antibacterial and synergy of berberines with antibacterial agents against clinical multi-drug resistant isolates of methicillin-resistant *Staphylococcus aureus* (MRSA). *Molecules.* 17 (9), 10322–30.

The microcirculation: a new frontier in cardiovascular phytotherapy

Kerry Bone

We receive nearly all our tissue nourishment and oxygen via the circulation of blood. The common view is that our circulatory or cardiovascular system consists of veins, arteries and the heart. Hence, all circulatory health problems are seen to arise from malfunctions of these key structures of the macrocirculation. But missing from this perspective is any consideration for the largest, and most neglected, part of our circulatory system. This is the microcirculation, the part that actually does the job of tissue nourishment. Allied to, and intimately connected to, the microcirculation is the concept of vascular endothelial function.

Gaining new insights into this overlooked topic can transform the way many patients are treated, including not only those with just circulatory problems, but an extraordinarily wide range of other common diseases as well. There is abundant clinical evidence that herbs and plant foods can play a key role in maintaining microcirculatory and endothelial health. In fact, at present there is much more comprehension of the benefits of plants in this context than for drugs.

A recent scientific review of the microcirculation observed (Wiernsperger and Rapin 2012):

> *'The difficulty of accessing microcirculation in view of the extremely small dimensions of these vessels has been by far the principal reason why this enormous anatomical entity has been essentially neglected for decades ... With very few exceptions, pentoxifylline and the antidiabetic metformin, no specific*

treatments have been developed for treating disorders at the microcirculatory level.'

What is the microcirculation?

The microvascular bed is an anatomical entity comprising countless small arterioles, capillaries and venules. Tissues such as the retina of the eye and the glomeruli of the kidney are particularly rich in microcirculation, because of their specific functions. The health of the microcirculation determines the blood supply and nutrient flow to all our vital tissues, but especially to vulnerable structures such as the long nerves that flow out of our spinal column to our limbs. Hence with diabetes, which damages the microcirculation, these tissues are specifically affected, namely as retinopathy, nephropathy and neuropathy. These come under the general heading of diabetic microangiopathy, which is the best known expression of microcirculatory disease.

The vascular endothelium

The vascular endothelium is the delicate monolayer of cells lining all blood vessels. It regulates the contractile and proliferative state of underlying smooth muscle cells and the interaction of the blood vessel wall with the circulating blood (eg as the gateway to immune cells, the process of haemostasis etc) (Wiernsperger and Rapin 2012). The myriad of tiny vessels throughout the body means the microcirculation contains the most significant proportion of the endothelial surface of the vascular bed. Hence, much of the understanding and implications of endothelial dysfunction are relevant to the consideration of microcirculatory health.

Microvascular physiology

The small arteries and arterioles dilate or contract to maintain a constant flow of blood to the microvascular bed (Wiernsperger and Rapin 2012). Capillaries are also able to regulate their flow by transmitting signals to upstream controlling arterioles. A multitude of factors influence the contraction or relaxation of arterioles (such as innervation, insulin, melatonin, blood viscosity and metabolites), but a key factor is nitric oxide (NO). In addition to this arteriolar control of capillary blood flow, other considerations are at play in determining the effective flow of blood through the capillaries. These include the haematocrit, blood viscosity and red blood cell deformability/aggregation.

Erythrocytes are biconcave-shaped elements that have an axial diameter usually above the internal capillary diameter. Thus, they must elongate to cross the tube: red cell deformability is therefore a crucial parameter for normal capillary flow, as illustrated by the vascular pain crisis in sickle cell anaemia patients (Wiernsperger and Rapin 2012).

Microvascular function and disease

According to a key review (Wiernsperger and Rapin 2012):

> *'The fundamental role of microvessels is to supply target tissues with oxygen and nutrients; therefore it appears logical that microvascular disorders will impact on tissue function, given the close coupling between flow and metabolism.'*

The review then goes on to list a range of diseases linked to microvascular dysfunction. These are overweight/obesity, diabetes, hypertension, low birth weight, sleep disorders, Alzheimer disease, gout, erythromelalgia, venous insufficiency, lupus, haemochromatosis, high ferritin, cardiometabolic syndrome, non-alcoholic steatotic hepatitis, polycystic ovary syndrome, gestational diabetes, acromegaly, rheumatoid arthritis, scleroderma, Behcet disease, hyperdynamic circulation, myocardial infarction, stroke, β-thalassaemia and HIV. But even this extensive list is incomplete. Based on the current literature we can credibly add the following diseases and applications: liver disease in general, kidney disease, neuropathies/neuralgias, restless legs syndrome, osteoarthritis (OA), retinal diseases, poor healing of any tissue, intervertebral disc damage, recovery from ischaemic damage, anti-ageing, athletic performance and cancer (especially for damage caused by conventional treatments).

OA and the microcirculation

One review suggested there is mounting evidence that a microvascular pathology plays a key role in the initiation and/or progression of OA (Findlay 2007). Disruption of microvascular blood flow in subchondral bone may reduce nutrient diffusion to the articular cartilage. Specifically, ischaemia in subchondral bone due to microthrombi may produce osteocyte death, bone resorption and articular damage. Another slightly earlier review suggested that vascular disease in subchondral bone may accelerate the OA process (Conaghan *et al.* 2005). This is either through reducing cartilage nutrition or (as per above) via direct ischaemic effects on bone, depending if cartilage damage is the primary or secondary inflammatory event in OA. Bone marrow lesions, linked to a poorer prognosis for knee OA, could be secondary to vascular events. Hence, regardless of what initiates OA (more relevant for prevention), vascular disease is also suggested to be highly relevant to its progression.

Heart disease and microcirculation

Coronary microvascular dysfunction is under intense investigation because of the growing awareness of its importance. For example, in patients with chest pain with a normal angiogram, coronary flow reserve (a measure of microvascular health) was a comprehensive indicator of cardiovascular risk (Lee *et al.* 2010). This was a study in 354 patients experiencing angina or angina-like chest pain.

The liver and microcirculation

There are major changes in the microcirculation in the liver with age. These include increased endothelial cell thickness and reduced numbers of pores (fenestrations). This is thought to contribute to dyslipidaemia, vascular disease, liver degeneration and poor drug metabolism (Le Couteur *et al.* 2005, 2008).

An article in the newspaper *The Australian* in 2006 by journalist Jill Margo noted the following about this research:

> *'Australian researchers have made a discovery that could prove beneficial to millions of older people. Through identifying how an ageing liver is starved of oxygen, they believe they may have uncovered an important factor in susceptibility to age-related diseases, including coronary artery diseases and nervous system disorders such as Parkinson's.... What they found had never been described before. They discovered that with age, tiny blood vessels in the liver undergo microscopic changes that can potentially translate into major diseases. Associate professor David Le Couteur, a geriatrician and clinical pharmacologist at the Canberra school, says a young, healthy liver has unique blood vessels. Unlike vessels anywhere else in the body, they are very thin and full of holes and look rather like the wire mesh in flyscreen. This mesh allows oxygen being carried in the blood to pass effortlessly into the liver cells where it is used to fuel metabolic processes. With age, Le*

Couteur says this fine mesh-like structure changes dramatically. The vessels thicken, the holes close off and an underlying basement membrane develops. This means less oxygen can get through and that the liver cells have less oxygen to do their metabolic work (including processing toxins)... The researcher's theory suggests that in old age these substances (toxins) can bypass the liver and deposit themselves elsewhere in the body where they can cause harm. Some fats may, for example, accumulate in coronary artery while a particular family of toxins might travel to the brain where they congregate and later manifest, perhaps as Parkinson's disease.'

Diabetic microangiopathy

Diabetic microangiopathy is directly linked to hyperglycaemia, and can be detected in people with only marginally raised blood glucose levels (Wiernsperger and Rapin 2012). A popular theory focuses on post-prandial hyperglycaemia: meals can interfere with normal blood vessel function even in healthy people. Inadequate eating (fat and/or sugar-rich meals) can, over time, damage the endothelial cells lining the micro-circulation (Wiernsperger and Rapin 2012).

As mentioned previously, type 2 diabetes (T2D) causes microvascular disease. But there is a growing school of thought that microvascular dysfunction is the fundamental cause of insulin resistance, leading of course to T2D (Wiernsperger and Rapin 2012). For example, retinal vascular calibre is one of several surrogate measures of microvascular dysfunction. A meta-analysis including more than 44,000 individuals found obesity was significantly linked to narrower arteriolar and wider venular calibres (Boillot *et al.* 2013). Another study concluded (Muris *et al.* 2012):

'These data indicate that various estimates of microvascular dysfunction were associated with incident T2DM and, possibly, impaired fasting glucose, suggesting a role for the microcirculation in the pathogenesis of T2DM.'

Endothelial function and disease

Closely allied to microcirculatory dysfunction is poor endothelial health. It is now thought that the initiating event in atherosclerosis is endothelial damage. Hence, the focus on endothelial dysfunction at present is its ability to predict arterial (large vessel) disease and the risk of a cardiovascular event (heart attack or stroke). Endothelial function can be measured by a number of techniques, including flow-mediated dilatation (FMD) and peripheral arterial tonometry (PAT), also known as the reactive hyperaemia index (RHI) (and sometimes called RH-PAT (Reriani *et al.* 2010). The former tests endothelial function in large conduit blood vessels, but the latter tests such function in small arteries and the microcirculation.

A recent review concluded that traditional cardiovascular (CV) risk factors based on the Framingham study do not adequately predict future CV events (Reriani *et al.* 2010). RH-PAT as a non-invasive measurement of endothelial function is emerging as a promising tool in CV risk prediction. Improvements in endothelial function have recently been linked to improved CV morbidity and mortality. A poor RHI also has been linked to the presence of vulnerable plaque, which is more likely to rupture and cause an acute CV event.

Erectile dysfunction (ED) in an otherwise healthy man is a warning sign of poor vascular endothelial health. In particular, endothelial nitric oxide production is typically impaired (Bone and Mills 2013).

Herbs and plant foods that benefit microcirculatory and endothelial health

The bilberry (*Vaccinium myrtillus* L.) (and here we could probably substitute the blueberry (*Vaccinium corymbosum* L.) as a less active alternative) has a long-held reputation for benefitting vision, and a significant part of this comes from its support of the microcirculation. For example, in open trials, bilberry extract improved symptoms caused by decreased capillary resistance (microvascular bleeding, bruising and faecal occult blood) (Piovella *et al.* 1996), reduced the microcirculatory changes induced by cortisone therapy in patients with asthma and chronic bronchitis (Carmignani 1983) and improved diabetic retinopathy with a marked reduction or even disappearance of haemorrhages (Orsucci *et al.* 1983). Post-operative complications from surgery of the nose were reduced in patients who received bilberry extract administered for 7 days before and 10 days after surgery, probably because of its benefits for the microcirculation (Mattioli *et al.* 1996). In placebo-controlled trials, bilberry extract improved early phase diabetic retinopathy (Repossi *et al.* 1987).

Garlic (*Allium sativum* L.) (particularly as the fresh-crushed raw clove or as an allicin-releasing powder) is good for both the microcirculation and microcirculatory flow. For example, in a controlled clinical trial a single 900 mg dose of garlic powder significantly increased capillary skin perfusion by 55 per cent (Jung *et al.* 1991). Another study found that garlic powder (600 mg/day) administered for 7 days increased lower limb blood flow by approximately 15 per cent (Anim-Nyame *et al.* 2004).

Two controlled trials have investigated the activity of gotu kola (*Centella asiatica* (L.) Urb.) actives (triterpenoids) in patients with microvascular damage due to diabetes. The largest trial involved 100 patients with or without neuropathy, and compared the extract with placebo over 12 months and also 40 healthy controls (Incandela *et al.* 2001). The herbal actives were significantly more effective at improving microcirculatory measures and oedema. A smaller trial in 50 patients compared a similar dose of gotu kola actives to placebo or no treatment for 6 months (Cesarone *et al.* 2001). There was significant improvement in the active treated group in measures linked to microscopic vascular damage, including capillary permeability.

Clinical studies of ginkgo (*Ginkgo biloba* L.) in retinal problems best illustrate its positive effect on microcirculation. For example, improved retinal artery and capillary flow rates have been observed (Chung *et al.* 1999, Huang *et al.* 2004), which probably would explain its effect on improving vision in patients with glaucoma (Quaranta *et al.* 2003), since glaucoma results in poor blood flow to the retina. In earlier research, a single dose of standardised ginkgo extract (112.5 mg) resulted in a significant increase in blood flow in nail capillaries in healthy volunteers (Jung *et al.* 1990). Another study demonstrated increased blood flow to the forearms of volunteers (Mehlsen *et al.* 2002). These studies confirm the ability of ginkgo to enhance microcirculatory flow.

Numerous clinical trials using doses of between 100 and 150 mg/day of OPCs from grape seed (*Vitis vinifera* L.) have demonstrated a beneficial effect on capillary resistance and capillary permeability (Morgan and Andrews 2007). For example, 100 mg/day of OPCs was administered to elderly patients with capillary fragility. Very good results were achieved in 67 per cent, good in 17 per cent and moderate in 13 per cent.

There are several studies suggestive of cocoa's (*Theobroma cacao* L.) positive effect on the microcirculation and endothelium. In a clinical trial, the impairment of endothelial function caused by a glucose challenge was reduced by dark chocolate, but not white chocolate (Grassi *et al.* 2012). Dark chocolate reduced endothelial dysfunction in breath-hold divers (Theunissen *et al.* 2013).

The beetroot (*Beta vulgaris* L.) is one of the richest sources of dietary nitrate. It is now realised that a specific pathway in the body can make nitric oxide from dietary nitrate: the nitrate-nitrite-nitric oxide pathway (Morgan 2013). This has profound implications for microcirculatory and endothelial health, and for regulating blood pressure.

Green tea (*Camellia sinensis* L.) for 2 weeks improved forearm endothelial dysfunction in smokers (Oyama *et al.* 2010). There was a significant increase in plasma nitric oxide. Green tea (4 weeks) improved flow mediated dilatation (FMD) (from 5.7 ± 2.7% to 8.7 ± 3.5%) in patients with chronic kidney disease (Park *et al.* 2010).

Insights from the Indian Paradox also point to other herbs that might be beneficial for microcirculatory and endothelial health. Briefly put, the prevalence of T2D in India is relatively high and with poor glycaemic control (average HbA1C 9.2 per cent). Yet eye complications (such as retinopathy) are only 16.6 per cent (Mohan *et al.* 2013), compared to Europe, Japan, the US and Australia at around 30 per cent (Raman *et al.* 2009). Could it be that the many spices in the Indian diet, especially turmeric (*Curcuma longa* L.), cayenne (*Capsicum annuum* L.) and ginger (*Zingiber officinale* L.), support microcirculatory health? The physiomedicalists described ginger as a 'diffusive stimulant', directly pointing to its effect on the microcirculation.

Based on the above, a 5-point dietary plan (with herbs such as gotu kola, grapeseed extract and ginkgo as additional treatments) can be recommended to patients with poor microvascular/endothelial health as follows:

- Boost dietary nitrate: green leafy vegetables, but especially beetroot as juice or a supplement.
- Increase cocoa intake: 85 per cent chocolate, 20 g/day.
- Increase berry anthocyanin intake: 50 to100 g/day of blueberries, strawberries, raspberries and blackberries.
- Raw crushed garlic: ½ to 1 clove/day.
- Increase herbs and spices: especially green tea (3 to 4 cups/day), turmeric and ginger.

A case history

A 61-year-old man presented with the main problem of declining kidney function. As well as having high blood pressure (controlled by multiple drugs), he also had type 2 diabetes, although this was well-controlled with just diet. Although his poor kidney function could have been caused by the diabetes, a medical specialist advised that some type of autoimmune damage to the glomeruli might be at play as well. In addition, tests showed that the tissue around his glomeruli exhibited a high degree of fibrosis, leading to a main diagnosis of arterionephrosclerosis. His glomerular filtration rate (eGFR) was quite abnormal at 35 and his plasma creatinine was elevated. His renal specialist had advised that he might be needing dialysis in 18 to 24 months.

The patient was recommended to follow the 5-point dietary plan above. In addition, he was prescribed tablets containing high doses of Echinacea root (for the autoimmune aspects), turmeric (anti-inflammatory and protective of the kidneys) and grapeseed, gotu kola and ginkgo for his microcirculation. As well, he was advised to take a high-dose fish oil supplement for its anti-inflammatory omega-3 fatty acids.

Five months later, the man had another blood test conducted by his medical specialist. To the surprise of both, his creatinine level had fallen by 33 per cent and his eGFR had risen to 51. His specialist commented that it was very rare for the eGFR to come back in this way, especially with his damaged kidneys. Normally it is a one-way decline. Eighteen months after the patient's initial presentation for herbal treatment his eGFR was normal at 74.

References

Anim-Nyame, N., *et al.*, 2004. Garlic supplementation increases peripheral blood flow: a role for interleukin-6 *The journal of nutritional biochemistry*, 15 (1), 30-36.

Boillot, A., *et al.*, 2013. Obesity and the microvasculature: a systematic review and meta-analysis. PLOS One, 8 (2), e52708.

Bone, K.M. and Mills, S.Y., 2013. *Principles and practice of phytotherapy: modern herbal medicine.* 2nd ed. UK: Elsevier, p. 330.

Carmignani, G., 1983. Le alterazioni del microcircolo di pazienti asmatici corticodipendenti e il loro trattamento. *Lotta contro la tuberce malattie polmonari sociali*, 53, 732-736.

Cesarone, M.R., *et al.*, 2001. Evaluation of treatment of diabetic microangiopathy with total triterpenic fraction of *Centella asiatica*: a clinical prospective randomized trial with a microcirculatory model. *Angiology*, 52(1-2), 49-S54.

Chung, H.S., *et al.* (1999) *Ginkgo biloba* extract increases ocular blood flow velocity. *Journal of ocular pharmacology and therapeutics*, 15 (3), 233-240.

Conaghan, P.G., Vanharanta, H. and Dieppe, P.A., 2005. Is progressive osteoarthritis an atheromatous vascular disease? *Annals of rheumatic diseases*, 64 (11), 1539-1541.

Findlay, D.M., 2007. Vascular pathology and osteoarthritis. *Rheumatology*, 46 (12), 1763-1768.

Grassi, D., *et al.*, 2012. Protective effects of flavanol-rich dark chocolate on endothelial function and wave reflection during acute hyperglycemia. *Hypertension*, 60(3), 827-832.

Huang, S.Y., *et al.*, 2004. Improved haemorrheological properties by *Ginkgo biloba* extract (Egb 761) in type 2 diabetes mellitus complicated with retinopathy. *Clinical nutrition*, 23 (4), 615-621.

Incandela, L., *et al.*, 2001. Treatment of diabetic microangiopathy and edema with total triterpenic fraction of *Centella asiatica*: a prospective, placebo-controlled randomized study. *Angiology*, 52 (2), 27-31.

Jung, E.M., *et al.*, 1991. Influence of garlic powder on cutaneous microcirculation. A randomized placebo-controlled double-blind crossover study in apparently healthy subjects. *Arzneimittelforschung*, 41 (6), 626-630.

Jung, F., *et al.*, 1990. Effect of *Ginkgo biloba* on fluidity of blood and peripheral microcirculation in volunteers. *Arzneimittelforschung*, 40(5), 589-593.

Le Couteur, D.G., *et al.*, 2005. The hepatic sinusoid in aging and cirrhosis: effects on hepatic substrate disposition and drug clearance. *Clinical pharmacokinetics*, 44(2), 187-200.

Le Couteur, D.G., *et al.*, 2008. Old age and the hepatic sinusoid. *Anatomical record* (Hoboken, 291(6)), 672-683.

Lee, D.H., *et al.*, 2010. Coronary flow reserve is a comprehensive indicator of cardiovascular risk factors in subjects with chest pain and normal coronary angiogram. *Circulation journal*, 74(7), 1405-1414.

Mattioli, L., Dallari, S. and Galetti, R., cited in Morazzoni, P. and Bombardelli, E., 1996. *Vaccinium myrtillus* L. *Fitoterapia* , 67(1), 3-29.

Mehlsen, J., *et al.*, 2002. Effects of a *Ginkgo biloba* extract on forearm haemodynamics in healthy volunteers. *Clinical physiology and functional imaging*, 22 (6), 375-378.

Mohan, V., Shah, S., Saboo, B., 2013. Current glycemic status and diabetes related complications among type 2 diabetes patients in India: data from the A1chieve study. *Journal of the association of physicians of India*, 61(1), 12-17.

Morgan, M. and Andrews, C., 2007. *Nutritional perspective*, 26, 1-3.

Morgan, M., 2013. Beet, Greens and herbs for health and vitality. *Nutritional perspective*, 38, 1-7.

Muris, D.M., *et al.*, 2012. Microvascular dysfunction is associated with a higher incidence of type 2 diabetes mellitus: a systematic review and meta-analysis. *Arteriosclerosis, thrombosis, and vascular biology*, 32 (12), 3082-3094.

Orsucci, P.L., *et al.*, 1983. Trattamento della retinopatia diabetic con antocianosidi Indagine preliminare. *Ann ottal clin ocul*, 5, 377-381.

Oyama, J., *et al.*, 2010. Green tea catechins improve human forearm endothelial dysfunction and have antiatherosclerotic effects in smokers. *Circulation journal*, 74 (3), 578-588.

Park, C.S., *et al.*, 2010. Green tea consumption improves endothelial function but not circulating endothelial progenitor cells in patients with chronic renal failure. *International journal cardiology*, 145 (2), 261-262.

Piovella, C., *et al.*, cited in Morazzoni, P. and Bombardelli, E., 1996. *Vaccinium myrtillus* L. *Fitoterapia*, 67 (1), 3-29.

Quaranta, L., *et al.*, 2003. Effect of *Ginkgo biloba* extract on preexisting visual field damage in normal tension glaucoma. *Ophthalmology*, 110 (2), 359-362.

Raman, R., *et al.*, 2009. Prevalence of diabetic retinopathy in India: Sankara Nethralaya diabetic retinopathy epidemiology and molecular genetics study report 2. *Ophthalmology*, 116 (2),311-318.

Repossi, P., Malagola, R. and de Cadihac, C., 1987. The role of anthocyanosides on vascular permeability in diabetic retinopathy. *Ann ottal clin ocul*, 113 (4), 357-361.

Reriani, M.K., Lerman, L.O. and Lerman, A., 2010. Endothelial function as a functional expression of cardiovascular risk factors. *Biomarkers in medicine*, 4 (3), 351-360.

Theunissen, S., *et al.*, 2013. Dark chocolate reduces endothelial dysfunction after successive breath-hold dives in cool water. *European journal of applied physiology*, 113(1), 2967-2975.

Wiernsperger, N. and Rapin J.R. 2012. Microvascular diseases: is a new era coming? *Cardiovascular and hematological agents in medicinal chemistry*. (10) 2, 167-183.

Premature Ovarian Failure (POF) and Infertility

Ruth Trickey

Premature ovarian failure (POF), resistant ovary syndrome (ROS), primary ovarian insufficiency, premature or early menopause are terms used to describe a group of related conditions characterised by failure of normal ovarian function, poor steroid hormone production, and lowered fertility potential. The estimated prevalence of POF is one in 1000 women aged 15-29 years and one in 100 women aged 30-39 years (Davis 2002). In the majority of cases the cause is unknown.

These conditions are not characterised by permanent cessation of ovarian function. Instead, folliculogenesis is intermittent, and ovulation (and pregnancy) can occur randomly (Kalantaridou and Nelson 2000). Steroidogenesis is similarly erratic such that symptoms of low oestrogen tend to relapse and remit.

The terminology and precise definitions used to describe these conditions are continuing to evolve. Premature ovarian failure (POF) is the favoured term. Resistant ovarian syndrome (ROS) is also used by some writers to define a sub-set of less serious symptoms associated with declining ovarian function. There is a suggestion that the condition should be renamed 'primary ovarian insufficiency' since this more fully characterises the intermittent nature of the complaint (Kalantaridou and Nelson 2000).

Some writers suggest that POF is actually a continuum of disorders that begin with increasingly poor ovarian function and terminate in permanent ovarian failure. This model describing intermittent and erratic ovarian function most closely reflects the clinical presentation of

POF, where women move from overt ovarian 'failure' to a functional ovarian state and back again in an unpredictable fashion (Popat *et al.* 2013).

This continuum has been described as having four clinically significant states:

Occult primary ovarian insufficiency:

- unexplained infertility, despite normal follicle stimulating hormone (FSH) levels
- failure to respond adequately to FSH therapy for ovarian stimulation for unexplained reasons

Biochemical primary ovarian insufficiency:

- unexplained infertility with elevated serum FSH level (usually taken on Day 2 of menstrual cycle)
- failure to respond adequately to FSH therapy for ovarian stimulation for unexplained reasons

Overt primary ovarian insufficiency (also known as resistant ovary syndrome):

- premature decline in ovarian function with elevated basal serum FSH levels in association with disordered menstrual cycles such as oligomenorrhoea, polymenorrhoea or metrorrhagia

Permanent ovarian failure:

- complete primordial follicle depletion
- eventually an irreversible state develops which is characterised by the presence of amenorrhoea, permanent infertility, and elevated menopausal gonadotrophin levels

The table opposite summarises the clinical and biochemical presentation.

Causes

Premature ovarian failure can be spontaneous or induced. Causative factors can be difficult to elucidate in all cases, but include:

Genetic defects largely involving the X chromosome or autosomal involvement

The most common genetic abnormality causing POF is Turner's syndrome.

OVARIAN CLINICAL SITUATION	MENSES	GONADOTROPHINS	FERTILITY
Occult insufficiency	Normal	Normal	Reduced
Biochemical insufficiency	Abnormal	Elevated	Reduced
Overt insufficiency	Abnormal	Elevated	Reduced
Premature ovarian failure	Absent	Elevated	Zero

Clinical Situations of Primary Ovarian Insufficiency and Premature Ovarian Failure (Popat et al. 2013)

Familial

The incidence of familial POF is reported to be around 4 per cent (Vujovic, 2009).

Autoimmune ovarian damage

About 20 per cent of women with POF are thought to have a co-existing autoimmune disorder (Goswami and Conway 2005).

Surgical treatment or radiotherapy or chemotherapy for malignancies

The effects of both radiotherapy and chemotherapy are dependent on age and ovarian reserve so that younger women are much more likely to resume ovarian function following either of these two interventions than older women (WsH Program 2010).

Environmental factors

Environmental factors include viral infections including mumps, Shigella, malaria and varicella. Endocrine disrupters, cigarette smoking, heavy metals, solvents, plastics, pesticides, industrial chemicals and various other toxins may also be capable of causing POF (Sharara *et al.*1998).

Enzyme deficiencies

Women with galactosaemia usually develop POF.

Diagnosis

A diagnosis of POF is made if a woman of less than 40 years of age has the following signs and symptoms (Kalantaridou *et al.* 1998, Davis 2002):

- amenorrhoea for four months or more
- low oestrogen levels
- an elevated FSH (confirmed by two to three FSH levels of >40 IU/L at least one month apart)
- poor rate of spontaneous pregnancy

When a chromosomal abnormality is detected, a diagnosis of POF can be made with certainty. Women with POF also have undetectable or greatly reduced levels of anti-Müllerian hormone (AMH) which is produced by the granulosa cells in the early stage of follicular development (La Marca *et al.* 2009).

Clinical findings

History may elicit conditions known to have a close association with POF, including autoimmune disease, or iatrogenic causes. Family history is important because POF is familial in some cases. Physical examination can be unremarkable, but signs of low oestrogen might be apparent, although these resolve with the return of ovarian activity. The ovaries in established POF are typically small and non-functional.

Biochemistry and imaging

- pregnancy test
- FSH, luteinising hormone (LH), oestradiol
- fasting glucose, electrolytes, and creatinine
- karyotype
- test for fragile X chromosome (FMR1 pre-mutation)
- thyroid-stimulating hormone (TSH)
- anti-thyroid peroxidase antibody
- serum adrenal antibodies
- bone density by dual-energy x-ray absorptiometry (DEXA) scan.

Management

The management of POF and related ovarian dysfunction depends on the life stage and desires of the woman. For young women not wishing to achieve a pregnancy, treatment with hormone therapy (HT) is the preferred option to improve symptoms associated with inadequate oestrogen levels and to reduce risk of osteoporosis later in life. Women with oligomenorrhoea and infrequent ovulation, even when asymptomatic for low oestrogen (hot flushes, vaginal dryness), experience prolonged periods of inadequate oestrogen levels since steroidogenesis occurs in conjunction with follicular development. These women are candidates for HT, especially when baseline DEXA shows osteopenia or osteoporosis. Non-medical options, while capable of managing symptoms of low oestrogen, do not protect bones against the rapid and premature bone density loss associated with absence of oestrogen and should not be recommended to osteopenic or osteoporotic women. All women should be given appropriate advice on the non-hormonal dietary, supplemental and life style factors that can be recruited to maintain bone health (Trickey 2011).

Fertility

Young women with POF should be offered counselling at diagnosis and given full information on the unpredictable nature of POF in terms of symptoms and fertility. Women wanting to conceive may respond more favourably to herbal management than to conventional medical options. The effectiveness of herbal treatment has not yet been thoroughly evaluated, however, and women need to be advised of this. Paradoxically, women who do not wish to achieve a pregnancy also need specific advice on contraceptive methods because oestrogen-containing combined oral contraceptive pills (COCP) will not necessarily prevent pregnancy. In these women conception has occurred while taking COCP (Rebar 2009), which appears to be related to the elevated gonadotrophin levels that initiate ovulation and negatively influence contraceptive effectiveness of COCP (Popat 2007).

Embryo cryopreservation, ovarian tissue cryopreservation and oocyte cryopreservation are usually offered to women where ovarian failure is foreseeable, such as when a woman is to undergo cancer treatments.

For the purposes of evaluation, a day 2 FSH level between 6 and 8 IU/L represents optimal ovarian function; while day 2 levels below 4 IU/L can indicate the presence of hormone (oestrogen) producing ovarian cysts. This can be a feature of POF because the poorly functioning ovary can produce anovular cysts in the presence of elevated FSH levels rather than normal functional ovarian follicles.

FSH levels in excess of 15 IU/L will typically result in poor conception rates or unsuccessful IVF treatments and IVF clinics with

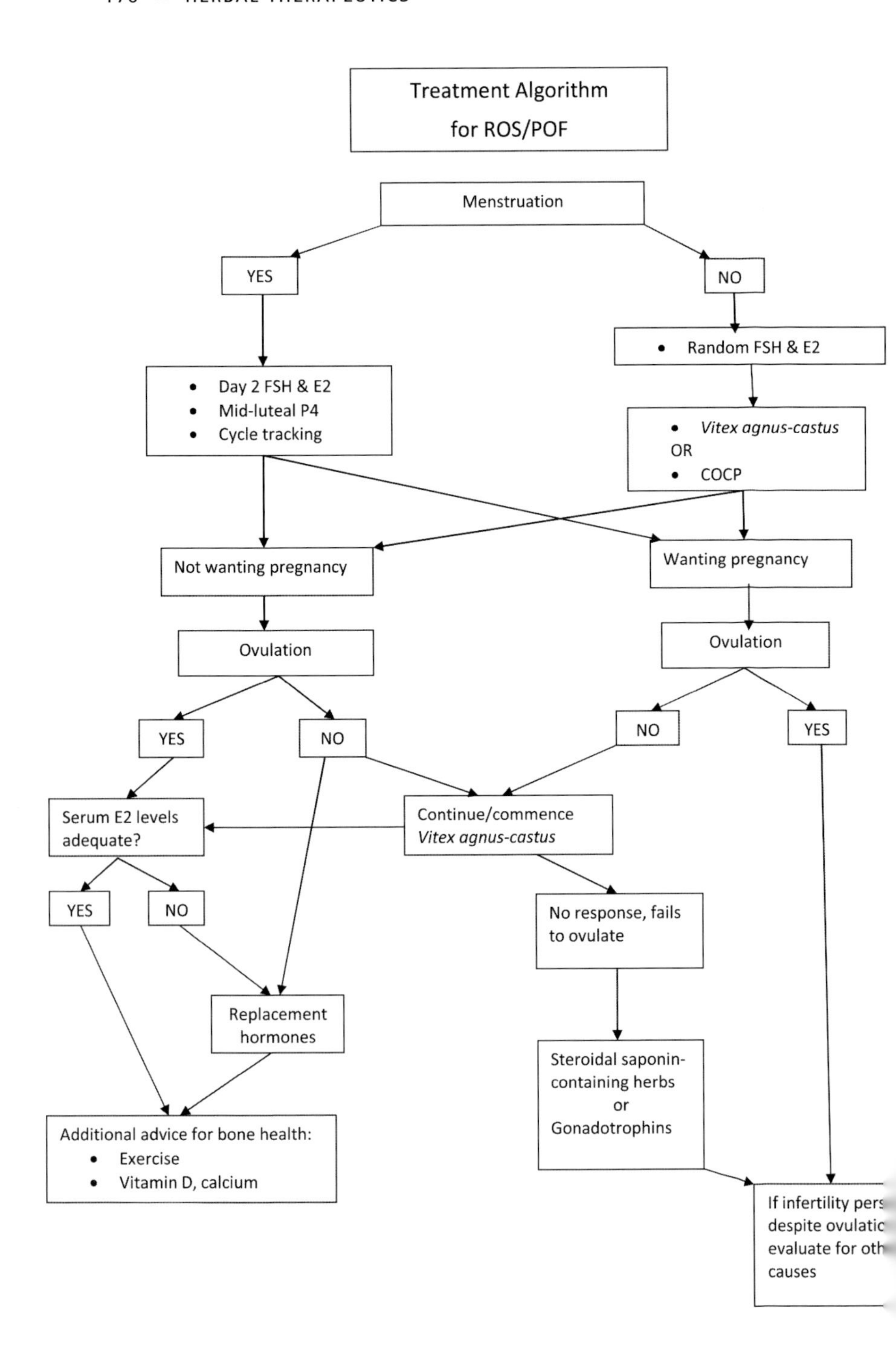
Treatment Algorithm for ROS/POF
Menstruation
YES
NO
Random FSH & E2
Day 2 FSH & E2
Mid-luteal P4
Cycle tracking
Vitex agnus-castus
OR
COCP
Not wanting pregnancy
Wanting pregnancy
Ovulation
Ovulation
YES
NO
NO
YES
Serum E2 levels adequate?
Continue/commence Vitex agnus-castus
YES
NO
No response, fails to ovulate
Replacement hormones
Steroidal saponin-containing herbs
or
Gonadotrophins
Additional advice for bone health:
Exercise
Vitamin D, calcium

expertise in the treatment of POF are likely to cancel cycles when FSH levels exceed their prescribed cut off limit.

Initiating normal ovarian function in women with POF is difficult. The only proven successful treatment is donor oocytes and IVF procedures (Laml *et al.* 2000). However, women with POF have ovaries that have become 'resistant' to the effects of not only endogenous, but also exogenous gonadotrophins and typically respond poorly to ovarian stimulation with these drugs. Thus response to assisted fertility with gonadotrophins is low due to poor ovum numbers at oocyte retrieval; or alternatively, failure of these oocytes to fertilise or mature.

In a medical setting, oestrogen therapy is often prescribed for one month as a means of checking ovarian reserve. This treatment also appears to trigger ovulation and improve the chance of pregnancy; perhaps by normalising LH level and preventing premature luteinisation of the remaining follicles (Popat 2007). Oestrogen therapy also improves endometrial development such that pregnancy can be sustained.

A treatment under review for the management of POF is *Vitex agnus-castus* L. The exact mechanism of action of this herb is unknown, but it appears in some way to improve ovarian receptivity to gonadotrophins. *Vitex* often results in lower FSH levels, and improved steroidogenesis and folliculogenesis. In instances where the follicular phase remains abnormally long, Vitex combined with steroidal saponin-containing herbs is a reliable strategy. These can be commenced in the early follicular phase, typically day 2, and ceased 2 days prior to anticipated ovulation. Alternatively, they can be prescribed all cycle.

Herbal protocols for treating POF

Occult and biochemical primary ovarian insufficiency; resistant ovary syndrome:

Women with ROS and POF can respond to *Vitex agnus-castus*. The herb is given alone to try to achieve a spontaneous pregnancy, or in combination with gonadotrophins during assisted reproductive technology cycles (ART) after discussion with the treating fertility specialist.

Women not undergoing ART who have a follicular phase longer than 21 days can also be given steroidal saponin-containing herbs from day 2 to day 12 of the menstrual cycle (pulsed steroidal saponins) as an attempt to induce ovulation.

Patients undergoing IVF who are being given high doses of gonadotrophins do not require pulsed steroidal saponins; however uterine tonics (see below) seem to be helpful to prevent the dyssynchronous endometrial development that can occur with high dose gonadotrophins.

A crude method of evaluating endometrial quality is to measure endometrial thickness; ideally 8 mm mid-cycle. A thin endometrium is indicative of low steroid hormone levels and indicates the need for uterine tonics in conjunction with *Vitex agnus-castus*. Possible candidates are dang gui (*Angelica sinensis* (Oliv.) Diels), peony (*Paeonia lactiflora* Pall.), rehmannia (*Rehmannia glutinosa* (Gaertn.) DC.) and shatavari (*Asparagus racemosus* Willd.).

Permanent ovarian failure:
Due to relapsing and remitting nature of POF; and because it is difficult to establish when an irreversible state has developed, a woman can be offered herbal intervention with this presentation. Women treated with *Vitex* have achieved successful pregnancies despite persistent amenorrhea, FSH levels well above 40 and symptoms such as hot flushes. However, when a woman with apparent permanent ovarian failure has been treated with herbs for 3 months or more without response there is little likelihood that ovarian function will resume.

Case History 1

Infertility following treatment for B cell lymphoma

A 34 year old year old woman who had had previous treatment for B cell lymphoma, with high dose cyclophosphamide, stem cell transplant and excision of mediastinal mass was referred by her fertility specialist. Her referral letter stated: 'There is some resurrection of ovarian function but we have been unable to freeze eggs or have a successful IVF cycle.' The patient reported that menstruation resumed about 11 months after completion of radiation therapy, but that this was erratic with a lighter flow than previously. Although some follicular development was evident on ultrasound, she had not conceived during 12 months of trying for a spontaneous pregnancy; nor ovulated with gonadotrophin stimulation. A day 2 FSH taken before her first consultation was 46 IU/L.

She commenced on *Vitex angus-castus* (Ze 440, 60% ethanol m/m, drug-extract ratio 6–12:1, standardised to casticin) and cycle tracking showed ovulation and good levels of progesterone during the mid-luteal phase. She reported her menstrual flow as looking like pre-treatment flow. For the three following cycles on *Vitex angus-castus* her day 2

FSH was between 20-26 IU/L, she had normal thickness endometrium, was producing ovarian follicles each month and her cycle length was normal. Disappointingly, she did not conceive. The following cycle it was decided to try another IVF cycle because her day 2 FSH was in the desirable range at 6.8 IU/L.

This cycle was unsuccessful, despite remaining on *Vitex angus-castus* and gonadotrophins simultaneously. She was also given a herbal mix containing peony (*Paeonia lactiflora*), withania (*Withania somnifera* L.), rehmannia (*Rehmannia glutinosa*), black haw (*Viburnum prunifolium* L.), shatavari (*Asparagus racemosus*) as a uterine tonic. Another cycle on IVF was attempted (day 2 FSH 3.2 IU/L), but as often happens when women have POF, low levels of FSH are indicative of an ovarian cyst, and the cycle was abandoned because of this.

At follow up review it was decided to attempt spontaneous pregnancy for another two cycles with the expectation of a better outcome because day 2 FSH was now in the normal range. This young woman went on to achieve a successful and healthy pregnancy during the second of these cycles.

Case History 2

Spontaneous POF

Thirty six year old G3P1M2 has been diagnosed with POF. She has had one miscarriage, followed by a successful spontaneous pregnancy at 33 and another miscarriage after this pregnancy. Her menstrual cycle for the past 2 years following the birth had been uncharacteristically erratic, and 10 months ago she developed hot flushes and periods of amenorrhoea exceeding 3 months. Evaluation by a fertility specialist revealed random FSH 45 IU/L and AMH <1; however, following menstruation her day 2 FSH was 10 IU/L and IVF was attempted. One follicle developed, but oocyte retrieval was unsuccessful. A subsequent IVF cycle resulted in 3 oocyte retrieval, but none of these fertilised and she was referred for herbal treatment.

She was started on *Vitex agnus-castus* (Ze440) 1 tablet every morning in conjunction with a number of nutrients to attempt to improve oocyte quality. In addition, because of the long follicular phase, she was prescribed Tribulus Forte, MediHerb (*Tribulus terrestris* 13.5g, standardised to 110 mg furostanol saponins as protodioscin) 1 BD from day 2-12 of menstrual cycle.

The following day 2 FSH was 24 IU/L so IVF was not attempted. Her fertility specialist recommended that she try for a spontaneous pregnancy over the next two cycles. To facilitate this, she also commenced a herbal formulation containing withania (*Withania somnifera*), shatavari (*Asparagus racemosus*), dang gui (*Angelica sinensis*), peony (*Paeonia lactiflora*) and rehmannia (*Rehmannia glutinosa*).

Ultrasound imaging at day 12 showed 7 mm endometrium, but no follicles. In addition, the patient was experiencing hot flushes, indicating that ovarian function was in decline. The ratio of *Asparagus racemosus* (Shatavari) was increased in her mix so that she was taking a weekly dose of 60 mL which reduced her hot flushes. Despite these treatments; however, ovarian function did not resume but menstruation occurred after 49 days. The following cycle (day 2 FSH 23.6 IU/L), Tribulus was increased to 2 BD from day 2-12 and an 18 mm follicle formed by day 12. She failed to achieve a spontaneous pregnancy.

Day 2 FSH in the following cycle was 4.6 IU/L and she was started on an IVF protocol while taking *Vitex agnus-castus* (Ze 440) 1 in the morning. Tribulus Forte was ceased. The IVF cycle was aborted, however, when she was found to have an ovarian cyst. Following menstruation, day 2 FSH 17.5 IU/L it was decided to try *Vitex agnus-castus* (Ze 440) 1 in the morning with low dose gonadotrophins (Gonal F 100 IU). This resulted in two follicles and she will try for a spontaneous pregnancy during this cycle.

Comment

Of these patients, one achieved a successful pregnancy, while the other has not and may not do so. Less than one third of women with declining ovarian function achieve a successful pregnancy with herbal treatment and this should be discussed with women before they are offered this type of management.

The usual protocol is to attempt to normalise ovarian function (lower FSH readings, improved steroid hormone production and improved fertility):

Vitex agnus-castus (Ze440) 1 daily in the morning:

- without steroidal saponins if the follicular phase is < 21 days or
- with Tribulus Forte, MediHerb (*Tribulus terrestris* 13.5g, standardised to 110 mg furostanol saponins as protodioscin) 1 BD from day 2-12 of menstrual cycle

If FSH is below 15 IU/L, IVF can be attempted. *Vitex agnus-castus* should be continued and uterine tonics may be required throughout the IVF cycle, particularly when high doses of gonadotrophins are prescribed. Pulsed steroidal saponin-containing herbs should be ceased in cycles where gonadotrophins are to be prescribed.

References

Davis, S., 2002. Abstracts from the 10th world congress on the menopause. Berlin, Germany, June 10-14, 2002. *Climacteric*, 2 (5,S1), 1-230.

Goswami, D, and Conway, G.S., 2005. Premature ovarian failure. *Human reproduction update*,11, 391-410.

Kalantaridou, S.N. *et al.*, 1998. Premature ovarian failure. *Endocrinology and metabolism clinics of North America*, 27, 989-1006.

Kalantaridou, S.N. and Nelson, L.M., 2000. Premature ovarian failure is not premature menopause. *Annals of the New York Academy of sciences*, 900, 393-402.

La Marca, A. *et al.*, 2009. Table ESIGfRE--AR. Anti-Mullerian hormone (AMH): what do we still need to know? *Human reproduction*, 24, 2264-75.

Laml, T. *et al.*, 2000. Premature ovarian failure: etiology and prospects. *Gynecology endocrinology*, 14, 292-302.

Popat, V. *et al.*, 2013. *Ovarian insufficiency* [Online]. New York: Medscape. Available from: http://emedicine.medscape.com/article/271046-overview - showall [Accessed 01/05 2014].

Popat, V.P., and Nelson, L.M., 2007. Spontaneous primary ovarian insufficiency and premature ovarian failure'. *Medscape*

Program WsH., 2010. Premature ovarian failure (POF). Monash University, Melbourne: Women's Health Program.

Rebar, R.W., 2009. Premature ovarian failure. *Obstetrics and gynecology*, 113, 1355-63.

Sharara, F.I., *et al.*, 1998. Environmental toxicants and female reproduction. *Fertility and sterility*, 70, 613-22.

Trickey, R.E., 2011. Women, hormones and the menstrual cycle. Melbourne, Australia: Trickey Enterprises (Victoria) Pty Ltd.

Vujovic, S., 2009. Aetiology of premature ovarian failure. *Menopause international*, 15, 72-5.

Rheumatoid arthritis and other systemic connective-tissue diseases

Fred Fletcher Hyde

This article was originally published in the New Herbal Practitioner *in 1975. Common plant names and authority for Latin binomials have been included in the first instance.*

Part 1

The group of musculo-skeletal disorders known popularly as 'rheumatic complaints' account for more time lost from work than any other disease, apart from bronchitis. Although much research has been carried out, the causative factors and the mode of pathogenesis are still in some measure of doubt. The study of the processes associated with ageing may be relevant, especially with regard to the localised degenerative changes of osteoarthrosis (osteoarthritis). In osteoarthrosis there is degeneration of the articular cartilage in one or two larger joints, bony outgrowths are formed at the edges of the joint and loose bodies of calcified cartilage may form in the joints. Cysts becoming cartilaginous and later bony may be present: they are known as Heberden's nodes and have a hereditary tendency. The release of enzymes mainly acid protease, initiating inflammatory changes is thought to be related to an increase in the permeability of lysosomes with age.

Aetiology of rheumatoid arthritis

1. Auto-immune response

Rheumatoid arthritis and related diseases are characterised by the involvement of the body as a whole, in contrast to osteoarthrosis in which the symptoms are localised and not systemic. There are two main theories to account for the inflammatory changes in this condition. One is based on the immune response of certain cells which react with antigens present in connective tissue as if they were foreign antigens and thus initiate an inflammatory reaction. This is known as an autoimmune response and results in lysosomal activity liberating in the tissue such inflammatory substances as histamine, kinins, 5 – hydroxytryptamine and prostaglandins. There is subsequent increased vascular permeability, erosion of cartilage, proliferation of the synovial membrane with pain, swelling, and heat.

2. Exogenous factors

The other theory has been advanced by the discovery of virus antibody in rheumatoid arthritis and by the disease arising as a sequel to syphilis, gonorrhoea, tuberculosis, brucellosis and septicaemia. Workers in Minnesota testing cases for German measles antibody conclude that their data indicate that 'prior infection with rubella virus or a closely related virus may be the aetiological basis of rheumatoid arthritis' in certain persons (Deinard 1974).

Dr E.C. Barton-Wright puts forward the hypothesis that 'rheumatoid arthritis and osteoarthritis are caused by a deficiency of pantothenic acid' (Barton-Wright 1974). A molecular defect in the structure of collagen from arthritics may increase the resistance of the joint cartilage to mechanical stress (Nimni and Deshmukh 1973, Francis and Smith 1974).

3. Liver disease

The role of the liver in connective tissue disease has been reported by Long and James (1974) in a case of polymyalgia rheumatica. There was hepatic involvement and 'sub clinical hepatic dysfunction' may be associated with polymyalgia rheumatica (Long and James 1974). This connection of liver disease with polymyalgia rheumatica was confirmed by subsequent reports (Gibbs 1974, Dickson and Maldonado 1974).

4. Hereditary factor

There is a moderate prevalence of familial occurrence. The diathesis may not develop in the absence of other factors.

5. Endocrine factors
The disease affects women two or three times as frequently as men. The exacerbation of symptoms at the menopause and quiescence during pregnancy indicate hormonal involvement. It is rare in hyperthyroidism.

6. Age
The disease may affect any age group although the commonest age for onset is 40. In children it is named Still's disease.

7. Psychological factors
Emotional disturbance, anxiety and depression may precipitate or exacerbate the condition.

8. Dietary factors
The excessive ingestion of animal protein in any form is contraindicated and may aggravate the disease. Oxalic acid containing foods such as asparagus, tomatoes and rhubarb may contribute to the worsening of the condition. Green salads and fruit have a contrary effect and should be consumed liberally. Vitamin C plays an important role in the health of connective tissue and the B-complex, including Vitamin B15 present in yeast and wheat germ (Scholz 1974), is also necessary to maintain healthy joint structures. Vitamins A, D1 and D2 are recommended in joint affections (Braem and Khetoua 1974).

Part 2

Grouped in accordance with the probable aetiology, giving main clinical features and a selection of suggested herbal remedies to be administered according to the indications of the patient as a whole. Specific remedies are highlighted in bold.

Group A

Endogenous or metabolic
The predominant cause arising from within the body.

1. Rheumatoid arthritis
A polyarthritis, affecting the smaller peripheral joints of hands and feet first, with general malaise and loss of weight. There is pain and inflammation; effusions may affect larger joints e.g. knee and elbow. Muscle wasting, anaemia and mononeuropathy, e.g. carpal tunnel syndrome,

are common. Both liver function and intestinal absorption may be affected (Surala *et al.* 1965).

Treatment

Diet should include a liberal amount of Vitamin C. The following remedies have been administered, alone or in various combinations, according to the needs of the individual patient and the spectrum of therapeutic activity of the remedy selected (British herbal pharmacopoeia).

Celery (*Apium graveolens* L.), black cohosh (*Cimicifua racemosa* (L.) Nutt), meadowsweet (*Filipendula ulmaria* (L.) Maxim), wintergreen (*Gaultheria procumbens* L.), guaiacum (*Guaiacum officinale* L.), wild yam (*Dioscorea villosa* L.), willow (*Salix alba* L.), boldo (*Peumus boldus* L.), sarsaparilla (*Smilax spp.*), prickly ash (*Zanthoxylum spp.*), poison ivy (*Rhus toxicodendron* (L.) Kuntz).

2. Acute gouty arthritis

An inborn metabolic disorder, rarely found in women. In most cases the great toe is the first joint to be affected, the inflamed metatarso-phalangeal joint becomes excruciatingly painful: there is general fever, anorexia and a polymorph leucocytosis. The plasma uric acid is raised and chalky tophi may be deposited in the pinna. Alcohol in excess, or high purine foods, may initiate an attack.

Treatment

Apium graveolens, *Guaiacum officinale*, carrot (*Daucus carota* L.), ground elder (*Aegopodium podagraria* L.), *Filipendula ulmaria*, *Peumus boldus*, wild lettuce (*Lactuca virosa* L.), valerian (*Valeriana officinalis* L.), gravel root (*Eupatorium purpureum* L.).

3. Chronic gouty arthritis

A similar condition in which there is incomplete remission between attacks. Rheumatoid nodules may form. The response to uricosuric agents is slow.

Treatment

Autumn crocus (*Colchicum autumnale* L.).

4. Menopausal Arthritis

The increase of gonadotrophic hormones and reduction in the oestrogen and progesterone may precipitate rheumatoid arthritis. Increase in weight will aggravate early osteoarthrosis.

Treatment
Blue cohosh (*Caulophyllum thalictroides* (L.) Michx.), *Dioscorea villosa*, cramp bark (*Viburnum opulus* L.), liquorice (*Glycyrrhiza glabra* L.) (Cheng-chia *et al.* 1973, Cotteril *et al.* 1973), *Cimicifuga racemosa*, *Smilax spp.*, and chaste berry (*Vitex agnus-castus* L.).

5. Psoriatic arthritis
Arthritis in association with psoriasis is more erosive than rheumatoid arthritis, the terminal interphalangeal joints are usually involved and the nails are ridged and pitted. The toes may become red and thickened – 'sausage toes'. Pustular psoriasis may develop on the soles of the feet.

Treatment
Burdock (*Arctium lappa* L.) root, *Smilax spp.*, chickweed (*Stellaria media* (L.) Vill.), thuja, (*Thuja occidentalis* L.) and Vitamin C.

6. Polymyalgia rheumatica
Mainly affects the elderly, women more often than men. There is proximal joint and muscle pain with stiffness in mornings, referred to hips, shoulders or spine. A mild arteritis may be evident in sensitivity of the carotid artery to light pressure.

Treatment
Gaultheria procumbens, bogbean (*Menyanthes trifoliata* L.), hawthorn (*Crataegus spp.*), angelica (*Angelica archangelica* L.), *Zanthoxylum spp.*, *Guaiacum officinale.*

7. Ankylosing spondylitis
An inflammatory arthritis which affects the spine of younger persons, from 20–40 years of age, men much more frequently than women. It is insidious and may progress from low back or 'sciatic' pain to spinal immobility. May be associated with ulcerative colitis, psoriasis (Brewerton *et al.* 1974)) or rheumatoid arthritis in the presence of histocompatibility antigen HL-A 27 (Vischer 1974, Calin *et al.* 1974).

Treatment
Guaiacum officinale, Zanthoxylum spp., Dioscorea villosa, Menyanthes trifoliata, Filipendula ulmaria, yellow clover (*Melilotus officinalis* (L.) Pall), chamomile (*Matricaria recutita* L.) (Breinlich 1968).

8. Systemic lupus erythematosus
An acute systemic disease, mainly affecting young females and characterised by fever, anaemia, facial skin eruption and joint pains. Considered to be an auto-immune condition, involving the cardio-vascular system, the kidneys or the liver in a large proportion of cases. Unfavourable prognosis is associated with persistent proteinuria, C.N.S. involvement or uraemia.

Treatment
Dioscorea villosa, Peumus boldus, poke root (*Phytolacca Americana* L.), dandelion (*Taraxacum officinale* Spp.), *Valeriana officinalis.*

9. Scleroderma and systemic sclerosis
A disorder in which the collagen of the skin becomes dense and fibrosed. In scleroderma the face and thorax may be affected following an infect-ion. Women are the usual sufferers. The viscera may be involved.

Treatment
Colchicum autumnale (Lush 1974), bladderwrack, (*Fucus vesiculosus* L.), comfrey (*Symphytum officinalis* L.), Vitamin B12, *Peumus boldus, Glycyrrhiza glabra, Cimicifuga racemosa, Caulophyllum thalictroides, Zanthoxylum sp.*, hart's tongue (*Scolopendrium vulgare Sm*).

10. Polyarteritis nodosa
In this disease the intima of many arteries, small to medium in size, becomes necrosed and aneurysms may occur. The skin of the legs may appear mottled. There is fever and joint pain. Men of all ages are mainly affected. Thrombosis and asymmetrical neuropathy may develop.

Treatment
Crataegus spp., Filipendula ulmaria, mistletoe (*Viscum album* L.) (Vogel *et al.* 1968, Burgio and Ugazio 1974, Becker von *et al.* 1971, Sakurai *et al.* 1971), *Gaultheria procumbens, Guaiacum officinale, Stellaria media, Zanthoxylum spp.*

11. Sjogren's disease
In association with rheumatoid arthritis symptoms, the lachrymal and salivary glands are deficient in secretion. The latter may become enlarged. The dryness of the mouth and hoarse voice, together with joint pains and keratoconjunctivitis are characteristic of this uncommon disease which usually occurs after the menopause.

Treatment
Oregon grape (*Berberis aquifolium* Pursh), *Glycyrrhiza glabra*, *Dioscorea villosa*, *Caulophyllum thalictroides*, *Phytolacca americana*.

12. Dermatomyositis
An infrequent disorder in which there is inflammatory degeneration of voluntary muscles with dermatitis and oedema, particularly of the eyelids. This condition is often associated with malignancy. A purplish discolouration may appear on the extensor surfaces of the limbs and around the eyes. Joint pain is frequent but relatively mild.

Treatment
Phytolacca americana, *Thuja occidentalis*, *Viscum album*, *Melilotus officinalis*, *Guaiacum officinale*, *Viburnum opulus*.

A number of disorders of the metabolism and endocrine system are associated with arthritis. They include amyloidosis, chondrocalcinosis, ochronosis (a tyrosine metabolic abnormality); hypothyroidism, hyperparathyroidism and acromegaly. *Fucus vesiculosus* may be used in arthritis with hypothyroidism. *Dioscorea villosa* in arthritis with acromegaly.

Group B

Exogenous
Conditions in which some external factor, often microbial, plays a predominant role in aetiology.

1. Rheumatic fever
An acute condition, mainly in children and adolescents which is characterized by pain and swelling in two or more joints with pyrexia, night sweats, epistaxis and carditis with tachycardia. Rheumatic nodules may occur in knee or elbow joints. There is often a history of prior

pharyngitis or tonsillitis and the lesions may be due to immune reaction to group A haemolytic *streptococcus*. The arthritis migrates from joint to joint and leaves no deformity.

Treatment

May include *Filipendula ulmaria*, *Salix alba*, poplar buds (*Populus gileadensis* Rouleau), agrimony (*Agrimonia eupatoria* L.), balmony (*Chelone glabra* L.), *Cimicifuga racemosa*, echinacea (*Echinacea angustifolia* DC), *Gaultheria procumbens*, motherwort (*Leonurus cardiaca* L.).

2. Still's disease

A juvenile rheumatoid arthritis of unknown aetiology which affects girls more than boys. The lymph nodes and spleen are enlarged in a third of cases, there may be intermittent pyrexia with a maculopapular rash. The condition commonly resolves although some joint changes may persist.

Treatment

Filipendula ulmaria, *Populus gileadensis*, *Phytolacca americana*, *Menyanthes trifoliata*, *Scolopendrium vulgare*, *Berberis aquifolium*.

3. Acute pyogenic arthritis

Arising by blood-borne infection from a focal sepsis, often a wound, which has become invaded by *Streptococcus*, *Staphylococcus*, *E. coli* or other microbial organisms. Features include enlarged, inflamed joint with much pain and a fever.

Treatment

Arctium lappa root, *Echinacea angustifolia*, nasturtium (*Tropaeolum majus* (L.) Kuntze), *Populus gileadensis*, *Juniperus communis*, *Lactuca virosa*.

4. Tuberculous arthritis

A monoarticular condition affecting children mainly, the pain is often worse at night. During the gradual onset of the inflammation there is a wasting of muscles around the joint. There is evidence of a tuberculous focus elsewhere in the body.

Treatment

Echinacea angustifolia, elecampane (*Inula helenium* L.), *Populus gileadensis*.

5. Reiter's disease
A syndrome of arthritis with acute urethritis and conjunctivitis. A virus Bedsonia, transmitted during sexual intercourse, is recoverable from the serum. Formerly mycoplasmas were thought to be the main cause. Any joints may be involved but usually the feet and ankles are affected. Occurs mainly in young men.

Treatment
Apium graveolens, bearberry (*Arctostaphylos uva-ursi* (L.) Spreng), *Gaultheria procumbens*, *Menyanthes trifoliata*, *Filipendula ulmaria*, *Arctium lappa* root, *Taraxacum* Spp., juniper (*Juniperus communis* L.), *Eupatorium purpureum.*

6. Gonococcal arthritis
Displays symptoms similar to Reiter's disease, but may also show a maculopapular rash. The joint fluid yields gonococci. A history of prior urethritis over several weeks differentiates this condition from rheumatoid arthritis.

Treatment
Arctium lappa root, *Echinacea angustifolia*, *Juniperus communis*, *Filipendula ulmaria*, *Peumus boldus.*

A number of diseases may be associated with symptoms of joint inflammation due to invasion by the organism present in the primary focus. They include scarlatina, meningitis, brucellosis, leprosy; mumps, infective hepatitis, infectious mononucleosis; syphilis, dysentery, enteric fever; actinomycosis, aspergillosis and other fungal infections (Golding 1973).

For arthritis in association with infective hepatitis – *Peumus boldus*, *Chelone glabra* may be used; all microbial infections – *Echinacea angustifolia* may be used; leprosy – *Smilax* spp., *Centella asiatica* may be used; mononucleosis or mumps, *Phytolacca americana* may be used; viral disease – garlic (*Allium sativum* L.) and hypericum (*Hypericum perforatum* L.) may be used.

Group C

1. Neurogenic arthritis
Charcot's disease. An infection of the joints in association with neurological conditions such as tabes dorsales and syringomyelia. The trophic

disturbance leads to degeneration of the joint, with or without pain. This osteoarthrosis is known as Charcot's disease. A Charcot joint is an enlarged, hypermobile yet painless joint.

Treatment

Hops (*Humulus lupulus* L.), *Matricaria recutita*, chilli (*Capsicum minimum* L.), *Zanthoxylum spp.*, *Valeriana officinalis*, *Dioscorea villosa*, *Filipendula ulmaria*, Roman chamomile (*Chamaemelum nobile* (L.) All), *Thuja occidentalis*, *Lactuca virosa*, *Viscum album*.

While no attempt has been made to deal exhaustively with the rheumatic diseases nor with the plethora of remedies available to treat them, sufficient has been presented to indicate the complexity of the subject and the wide range of symptoms characteristic of these all too common afflictions. 'In spite of our increasing knowledge of relevant pathology and immunology the causes of these diseases are still largely unknown' (Cosh 1974), but long remission is frequently observed by the herbal practitioner, following his careful advice on regimen and diet and the administration of non-suppressive herbal remedies.

References

Barton-Wright, E.C., 1974 *Pharmaceutical journal* April 27.

Becker von, H. *et al.*, 1971 *Planta medica* 20 357.

Braem, T. and Khetoua, J.L., 1974 *Lichaam en Geest* 45. 759.

Breinlich, J., 1968 *Arzneimittel forsch.* 18 429.

Brewerton, D.A. *et al.*, 1974 1.c. 956.

British Herbal Pharmacopoeia (1974) Sections 1-3.

Burgio, G.R. and Ugazio A.G., 1974 *Lancet* 1 568.

Calin, A. *et al.*, 1974 1.c. 874.

Cheng-chia, L. *et al.*, 1973 *Chinese medical journal* 11 156. 13.

Cosh, J.A., 1974 *The practitioner* 213 519.

Cotteril, J.A. *et al.*, 1973 *Lancet* 1 294.

Dickson, E.R. and Maldonado, J.E. (1974) 1.c. 577.

Deinard, A.S. *et al.*, 1974 1 526.

Francis, M.J.O. and Smith, R., 1974, *Lancet* 1 841.

Gibbs, P., 1974 1.c. 352.

Golding, N.D., 1973 *Synopsis of rheumatic disease* 122–126.

Long, R. and James, O., 1974 *Lancet* 1 77–79.

Lush, B., 1974 *Lancet* 1 1054.

Nimni, M. and Deshmukh, K,. 1973 *Science* 181 751.

Sakurai, A. *et al.*, 1971 Foe. Sci. *Shiznoka* 6 63.

Scholz, H., 1974 *Naturheilpraxis* 324.

Surala, M. *et al.*, 1965 *Acta med.* Scand. 178 13.

Vischer, T.L., 1974 1.c. 1001.

Vogel, G. *et al..*, 1968 *Arzneimittel forsch.* 18 426.

Further reading

Fletcher Hyde, F., 1975 Rheumatoid arthritis and other systemic connective-tissue diseases, *New herbal practitioner*, 1(2), 55-62.

Reflecting on children's health over the last twenty-five years

Frances Hambly

My journey with herbal medicine and treating children has evolved over the years, we are always learning and expanding our knowledge, but some fundamentals stay the same, such as the importance of fever and diet and supporting the liver and digestive system.

It is interesting to reflect on what has changed over the years, as well as the things that stay the same – the recurrent themes that affect children during their childhood. Life has become more pressured for both parents and children, for example the explosion of technology into family life.

I remember measles being seen as an uncomplicated illness twenty-five years ago, and it still is if treated correctly. Childhood diseases do the rounds and have their own cycle appearing every few years. Whooping cough is a constant, measles is reappearing and now scarlet fever has emerged from the past. Teenagers and young adults often acquire childhood infectious diseases later in life when immunity from vaccinations has waned, for example when they are at critical stages in their education with exams and at university.

I have seen an increase in allergies and chronic illnesses. There is more asthma and eczema, and glandular fever, chronic fatigue syndrome and herpes viruses like shingles present themselves more frequently in young children. This all suggests an altered immune function in children. There are more children with learning disorders, attention deficit disorder (ADD) and autism spectrum disorder (ASD), more mental health issues like depression, and we have an epidemic of eating disorders. Poor muscle and bone development is becoming more prevalent and I also see more children and young people with thyroid issues.

Regardless of warnings over the last couple of decades on the overuse of antibiotics the drugs are still being administered for illnesses they will not be effective against. Disease causes fever and rashes which enable the body to cleanse itself and eliminate waste material. Suppression of these processes with antipyretics like paracetamol, antihistamines and steroids can lead to complications and long term chronic illness, especially in severe infection. The germ theory continues to instil fear into parents and health care workers

Fever is fundamental to a child's health and needs to be worked with, rather than against. Fever was once considered a healthy response to disease. The present attitude to treat even minor fevers with antipyretics is undermining the health of children's immune systems and causing repercussions in the long term. Seeing a sick child can be as distressing for the parents as it is for the child to be unwell. The wish to alleviate suffering as quickly as possible is only normal but antipyretics, rather like antibiotics are given by healthcare professionals as the only thing on offer to help allay the fears of parents.

A temperature is usually a sign of a robust immune system and in a healthy child fever poses little threat. The underlying health of the child is all important. Children, especially those under three years old, are at risk of febrile convulsions as their temperature control mechanism isn't fully developed. Certain illnesses like roseola provoke a particularly high temperature which can peak at 40.6 °C. Convulsions usually occur while the temperature is rising before parents realise their child is unwell. There is no evidence that fevers below 42 °C cause neurological damage, even in young infants. Despite advice to the contrary and evidence to say that they do not prevent febrile convulsions, antipyretics are still recommended for mild fevers. It is the child who is floppy and quiet with a normal or low temperature that would concern me, more than one who has a high temperature, who is alert and has enough energy to be vocal (NICE Guidelines 2007, WHO 1993).

Evidence indicates that fever is beneficial and it improves immune function. Fever increases B lymphocytes, thereby producing more antibodies, and activates T lymphocytes. A fever also inhibits the reproduction of certain microbes. Children who ran a fever during their first year were less likely to develop allergies later in childhood (Keoki Williams *et al.* 2004). I spend time explaining to parents why a fever should be seen as a good thing and its importance in illness, that illness is a cleansing mechanism and nature's way of eliminating toxins, and that fever is the response of a healthy body to infection.

Suppressing a fever unnecessarily with regular doses of Calpol is not in the best interest of the child and their developing immune system. I suggest only using paracetamol or ibuprofen if the child is in pain and where it can aid a restful sleep, but not to suppress a fever unnecessarily. Children given paracetamol might be more active and alert during their illness but this does not encourage them to rest nor does it speed up recovery. A fever can reduce the length and severity of illnesses and reduce the time a child is contagious.

Childhood illnesses should be viewed as stages in their development as well as in the maturation of their immune system. Children usually take a step forward in their development after a childhood illness. Acceptance of the germ theory creates fear and a frightened parent is a stressed parent. This stress is transferred to the child who in turn creates excess stress hormones which lower the effectiveness of the child's immune system (Donegan 2008).

As well as recognising the warning signs of severe illness most parents know when their child is not quite themselves. I encourage this innate intuition and nurture self confidence in parents' own abilities to support and care for a sick child by teaching basic nursing skills and equipping them with herbal alternatives to use at the first signs of illness. Parents are delighted when they manage to bring their child through an ear infection without antibiotics and paracetamol.

While a baby receives passive immunity via antibodies in its mother's milk, natural, usually lifelong immunity, is built up through exposure to germs and childhood diseases. Exposure to organisms at the right age allows the immune system to mature properly, producing antibodies appropriately. By adulthood if immunity to most diseases has been acquired naturally three to seven per cent of the immune system's capacity has been committed. The rest of the immune system is left free to deal with other challenges. With immunisation it has been estimated that this can rise to as much as 70 per cent (Dettman 1983).

Children are no longer exposed to micro-organisms at the optimum age and the immune system is not given the chance to produce antibodies naturally. The chances are that this leaves the child more susceptible to other infections, allergies and autoimmune diseases as they grow up. On top of this the effectiveness of the immune system is further compromised by the need for repeated boosters as passive immunity from vaccinations wanes alongside antibiotics, steroids, a poor diet, pollution and stress.

Diet has always been a big focus of my practice and I find that this underpins the way I work as allergies, food intolerances and autoimmune disorders become more of a problem. Processed foods contain an increasing amount of sugar as well as artificial sweeteners and wheat has emerged as an issue in younger children. A good diet is fundamental to a healthy immune system. An unprocessed diet full of natural, fresh, chemical free food consisting of vegetables and fruit, good quality protein and fats and oils will provide the essential building blocks for healthy growth and a robust immune system. A healthy gut and gut flora is key to absorbing and assimilating these nutrients. I encourage soaking and fermenting of grains, nuts and pulses; live yoghurt, sourdough and spelt bread, porridge made from soaked oats. Lacto-fermented foods provide beneficial bacteria to the gut which in turn aid digestion and guard against pathogens (Fallon 2009).

During any acute infection keep children on a light diet. Most children will lose their appetite, but if they are hungry give small amounts of soup or juice. Plenty of fluids are vital with a fever – breast milk, water or diluted juice, ideally including beetroot and carrot. Don't give any dairy produce or refined sugar. When the acute stage is over give plenty of vegetables, soup, broth, and fermented foods like yoghurt and kefir.

I encourage parents to introduce herb teas from an early age to get children used to the taste of herbs; these can be mixed with a bit of juice and given warm or cold. I tell parents about the medicinal uses of the herbs, spices and foods in their kitchen, for example how fantastic garlic is for infections. I give parents a list of things to have on hand, a basic dispensary for children with guidelines for doses. I use glycerites as much as possible with children, as well as aromatic waters. With tinctures I find drops allow for a more tailored dosage system with younger children and these can easily be administered in a little water or juice.

Essential oils used in the bath and in a nebuliser work fantastically well for coughs and colds as well as for relaxation. I use either of the echinacea species (*Echinacea angustifolia* DC. or *Echinacea purpurea* (L.) Moench) as an immune modulator across the board for many problems and elderberry is a tasty addition to an immune boosting mix.

Where the child is able to swallow tablets or capsules I will give andrographis (*Andrographis paniculata* (Burm.f.) Nees) with echinacea. Elderflower is wonderful for colds, catarrh and hay fever and when combined with lime flowers is a soothing diaphoretic in fever management. With children prone to febrile convulsions I would give catmint hourly. Spearmint is a good addition to herbal teas for taste as well as therapeutically. For coughs I will combine thyme with liquorice, elecampane and hyssop. To improve digestion and assimilation angelica root, common centaury, chamomile and dandelion root work effectively. Burdock, dandelion root and milk thistle aid elimination and detoxification. Chamomile, lemon balm, passionflower, skullcap and vervain work well for the nervous system, as well as having a positive effect on the digestive system.

Discussion about the immune system and fever leads to the vexed question of vaccinations. I discuss vaccinations with parents if they wish to do so. Babies are vaccinated for more and more diseases at a very young age, including *in utero* (Repevax is presently offered for whooping cough between 28-38 weeks of pregnancy), when they are going through a period of rapid brain growth and development, so it is worth considering the neurological effects vaccinations might have. I advise only to vaccinate if a child is 100 per cent, it is never worth vaccinating a sick child even if 'it's just a cold'.

If parents want to vaccinate but wish to minimise the side effects I suggest giving a good quality probiotic with an optimal immune boosting diet for at least one week before and two weeks after vaccination. To further optimise the child's health before vaccination antioxidants can be given via mum if baby is solely breast fed or as a supplement in the form of drops or tablet depending on the age of the child. A diet rich in vitamins A, C, D and E and essential fatty acids, particularly Omega 3 is important. I would give echinacea, dandelion root and milk thistle in tablet, tincture or glycerite form and nettles, cleavers and parsley piert as teas, glycerite or tincture for seven days from the day of the vaccine. A combination of Thuja 20 and Chelidonium 5 (25ml) tincture helps to counteract any adverse reactions. The dose for those aged 12 years and over is 10 drops twice a day the day before and two days after vaccination. I would only give 1-2 drops to babies and young children.

I try to make a plan that will work for the individual family. I like to spend time with the parents and child or children. It is insightful to see how the family dynamic works. Although illnesses have become more complicated, thankfully children still possess an innate ability to bounce back to health and instinctively often know what is good for them, especially when things are explained to them.

References

Dettman, G., 1983. *The dangers of immunisation.* Pennsylvania: Humanitarian Society.

Donegan, J., 2008. Fear. *The informed parent* [online]. Available from: http://www.jayne-donegan.co.uk/wp-content/uploads/articles/2008%20Fear%20website.pdf [Accessed 28 February 2014].

World Health Organization, 1993. The management of fever in young children with acute respiratory infections in developing countries. Available from: apps.who/iris/bitstream/10665/58266/1/WHO_ARI_93.30.pdf?ua=1 [Accessed 28 February 2014].

Fallon, S., 2009. *Nourishing traditions: the cookbook that challenges politically correct nutrition and diet dictocrats.* 2nd ed. US: New Trends Publishing.

NICE Clinical Guidelines, 2007. *Feverish illness in children: assessment and initial management in children younger than 5 years* (CG47). *NICE* [online]. Available from: http://guidance.nice.org.uk/CG47 [Accessed 06 May 2014].

Williams, L.K., *et al.*, 2004. The relationship between early fever and allergic sensitization at age 6 to7 years. *Journal of allergy and clinical immunology*, 113 (2), 291-296.

Further Reading

Hambly, P. and Buning, F., 1993. *Herbalism (headway lifeguides).* London: Hodder and Stoughton.

Hambly, F., 2004. *Herbal medicine for children.* Rochester: Amberwood Publishing.

McIntyre, A., 1992. *The herbal for mother and child.* Shaftesbury: Element Books.

Santich, R. and Bone K., 2008. *Phytotherapy essentials: healthy children, optimising children's health with herbs.* Queensland: Phytotherapy Press.

Posology in herbal medicine

Hein Zeylstra

This article was originally published in issue 4 (2) of the British Journal of Phytotherapy *(1995) and is reproduced here with the kind permission of the College of Practitioners of Phytotherapy. Common names and authority of Latin binomials have been included in the first instance.*

In contradistinction to the osteopath, chiropractor, or acupuncturist, the phytotherapist does not administer his or her treatment in the consulting room but in the form of medicine to be taken home by the patient. The treatment is determined by the act of prescription, which involves a decision on (a) which medicine or medicines to prescribe and (b) how much of this medicine should be taken. The phytotherapist is fortunate in being able to administer the same (plant) medicine in a variety of forms, including infusions, decoctions, hand, foot, or body baths, lotions, creams, suppositories, plasters, and, of course, tinctures. This article limits its discussion to the use of tinctures only. Even tinctures, however, can be prescribed in many different ways, for instance, a single tincture, a mixture of two or more, once a day, three to five times a day, before or after meals, and so on. The method of administration can be used to the advantage of the patient, but experience, knowledge, and mature reflection are needed to make the right choice.

This article will deal with a number of considerations related to the dosage and prescription of herbal tinctures in specific circumstances.

The average dose, maximum and minimum amount

The *British Pharmacopoeia* (BP), the *British Pharmaceutical Codex* (BPC) and the *British Herbal Pharmacopoeia* (BHP) often give a dose range instead of just one fixed dose. For instance, according to the *British Herbal Compendium* 1992, the dosage for gentian (*Gentiana lutea* L.) root is 1-4 ml of a 1:5 tincture (45 per cent) one to three times daily. This means that the practitioner has the choice of giving the patient between 1 and 12 ml of the tincture per day, allowing him or her considerable latitude. In calculating dosage, therefore, the following considerations should be taken into account:

- Frequency of administration. When a medicine is given only once a day, the single dose may be higher than when the same medicine is given two or three times daily.
- The age of the patient. A child usually gets a smaller dose, calculated according to age using set formulae. At the other end of the age spectrum, a frail 80-year-old is likely to need less medicine than someone of 35.
- Physical status and condition. An active young man weighing 170 lb is likely to need more medicine than an underweight woman of 100 lb. Individual susceptibility, either to medicine in general or to some medicines in particular. Whereas one person may respond hardly at all to x ml of a tincture, another may keel over at half that dose.
- Other medication, given either by the practitioner or by the patient's GP. This, clearly will affect the amount of tincture prescribed.

To conclude, the decision on how much of a particular herb to give rests entirely with the practitioner, but it should be based on a scientific evaluation of the case in hand.

One dose a day versus two to five doses a day

The decision on whether to give the patient a single dose or to administer the medicine more often takes into account factors such as:

- The fact that the medicine contains an active constituent which is slowly absorbed or metabolized, giving it a long-lasting effect for example, chaste berry (*Vitex agnus-castus* L.) or feverfew (*Tanacetum parthenium* L.). In this case administration once a day may be sufficient. The fact that the medicine contains constituents which are rapidly absorbed, metabolized, and/or excreted. Herbal medicines are normally taken three times a day, but in cases where the medicinal action may depend on, for instance, complex sugars such as those of echinacea, which enhance the activity of the immune system, the tinctures should be taken every two-and-a-half to three hours (five to six times a day), as the active constituents are broken down by the body within this time.

- The purpose of the medicine. A sleeping mixture, for instance, is usually given an hour or less before bedtime, not three times a day. Another case in point is the gargle, which should be used as often as possible, since it is the contact of the medicine with the inflamed mucous membrane which represents the principal mode of action. Gargling once a day in the morning for a few seconds to cure a sore throat is of no use.

Reflex actions

In phytotherapy we use the reflexes of the body to obtain actions in sites we cannot reach directly with our medicines. There are numerous everyday illustrations of the reflex principle: for example, one can observe that a dog whose 'armpit' is lightly stroked will suddenly jerk with his hind leg. The same criterion applies if one lightly strokes the mucous membranes of the gut: 'in sympathy' the other membranes of the body will react in a similar way. By giving small amounts of mucilages by mouth we therefore obtain a demulcent action on the membranes of the respiratory tract, urinary tract, etc. It is important to bear in mind that to elicit a reflex action the original stimulation of the nerve endings must be very gentle, as in the example of the dog given above. When eliciting the knee reflexes, we do not use a sledgehammer but a palpation hammer, and for the plantar reflexes we touch the sole lightly with a needle; we do not scratch it forcefully with a nail. The latter course of action would result in overstimulation of the nerve endings, leading to spasm or paralysis.

Thus, to treat an inflammatory condition of the lining of the stomach, in a case of gastritis or stomach ulcer, we administer large amounts of demulcents for their purely physical action in covering the inflamed mucous membrane, soothing it, isolating it from the contents and the juices of the stomach, and creating a favourable environment for healing; this would call for, say, marshmallow (*Althaea officinalis* L.) root, which contains around 30 per cent mucilage. Here, however, the sheer quantity of demulcent used means that any reflex action is blocked by overstimulation of the nerve endings.

If, on the other hand, a demulcent action is required in the respiratory tract, we need small doses which have no physical effect on the mucous membrane of the stomach but can trigger a reflex action elsewhere. The best way of obtaining this effect is to use herbs that contain small amounts of mucilage only, such as the aerial parts of *Althaea officinalis*, couchgrass (*Triticum repens* L.) or cornsilk (*Zea mays* L.). Again, this underscores the fact that, by using different parts of the same plant, we can achieve different effects or the same effect in different places.

Very small amounts versus large amounts: reversal of effects

It is common knowledge in phytotherapy that one can often obtain the opposite effect by using either a very small dose or a very large one (with regard to the former, we are still talking of material, not homoeopathic doses). A well-known example is the action of two herbs which in 'normal' doses act as bitters, but in very small doses have the opposite effect on the stomach. The two herbs are sweet flag (*Acorus calamus* L.) root and angelica (*Angelica archangelica* L.) root: 3-4 ml per day, divided into two doses taken about an hour before meals, will give the action of a reasonably strong bitter. In cases of hyperchlorhydria, however, we can use doses of 5-7 ml per week, and the production of hydrochloric acid will be moderately to strongly suppressed.

Another well-known example is that of valerian (*Valerian officinalis* L.). It is used by almost every practitioner as a sedative and relaxant, usually in doses of 25-50 ml per week, and, although the personal tolerance varies a great deal, these doses are generally well tolerated. However, if large doses, 100 ml or more, are prescribed for several weeks on end, a number of patients experience, in exaggerated form, the symptoms they originally sought help for, such as loss of orientation, severe restlessness, headaches, increased irritability, and so on.

In my view this phenomenon might well be explained by the reflex theory; the administration of small amounts will stimulate or sedate certain centra, but that of large amounts will block the possibility of a reflex and may produce the opposite effect to the one intended, be it a muscular, nervous, or psychotropic effect.

The time factor (chronopharmacy)

From the study of pharmacy and pharmacology it is known that the time of application of a drug often has a bearing on its efficacy. People who try to commit suicide with a mixture of barbiturates and alcohol, for example, often find that their attempt fails if it takes place in the evening (the time when suicide is most often attempted). However, suicide attempts carried out under similar circumstances early in the morning achieve a rate of mortality that is about 30 per cent higher, a phenomenon explained by the fact that the metabolic activity of the brain is greatest in the first few hours after waking up. For this reason, medicines that are supposed to work directly on the nervous system and/or the brain should be taken early in the day. *Vitex agnus-castus*, for instance, is usually given in a single dose first thing in the morning; its effect if it were taken later in the day would be about 30 per cent less.

Another important fact is that the activity of the kidneys slows down in late afternoon, and more or less stops during the late evening and night. Diuretics taken in the late afternoon or early evening will therefore produce hardly any increase in urinary output, whereas those taken early in the morning will have a maximal effect. Medicine prescribed for a kidney patient should thus be administered in the morning, again at midday, and then early in the afternoon if it is to be effective.

Similarly, medicine prescribed to aid digestion will take ½–1 hour to stimulate the ancillary organs of the digestive system. For this reason, bitters and similar preparations, most of which work by activating the nerve endings in the taste receptors located in the tongue, should be given about half to one hour before a meal, with the recommendation that they be slowly sipped over 15 minutes.

Medicines for the cardiovascular system should be given at around 10 am, when the heart is working at peak efficiency and then again either at lunchtime or as late in the evening as possible to take account of the fact that the heart slows down at around 4 pm (as well as at 4 am).

Before or after meals

From what has been said about bitters in the preceding section, it is obvious that they should always be given before a meal (an hour or so). The same applies to herbs such as lobelia (*Lobelia inflata* L.) and echinacea (*Echinacea* spp.), whose active constituents are quickly broken down by the digestive system; if taken after a meal they will remain in the stomach for a considerable time and hence be deactivated. Again, demulcents applied to the digestive tract, say in the case of a stomach ulcer, where the aim is to coat the lining with mucilage, must of course be given before food is ingested.

On the other hand, certain medicines such as prickly ash (*Zanthoxylum* spp.) may cause nausea or discomfort when given on an empty stomach, and these should be taken after a meal.

The toxic dose

With most herbal medicines there is a wide margin between the therapeutic and the toxic dose. Notable exceptions are those herbs containing tropane alkaloids such as belladonna (*Atropa belladonna* L.) thorn apple (*Datura stramonium* L.), and henbane (*Hyoscyamus niger* L.), where the dose ranges for the therapeutic and the toxic effect are extremely close. The best course of action in prescribing such medicines is to start with a subtherapeutic dose and then very slowly, either day by day or every two to three days, increase the dose until the therapeutic effect becomes noticeable, continuing until the maximum therapeutic effect has been achieved and the first side-effects occur. In the case of *Atropa belladonna*, *Datura stramonium*, and *Hyoscyamus niger*, this is usually a dry mouth; as soon as the patient notices this, he or she should reduce the dose slightly, and will then have achieved the optimum therapeutic dose.

It may also be that a herb administered in a single dose can be given in a much larger quantity than if prescribed on a regular basis. For instance, wormwood (*Artemisia absinthium* L.) can be given in a single dose of 5-7 ml first thing in the morning on an empty stomach if it is used as an anthelmintic or vermifuge, while if it is part of, say, a regular dose of bitters, no more than 1-2 ml should be given at a time. However, even a single dose of 5 ml may sometimes cause a headache.

Combinations

The art of combining herbal medicines is less simple than it appears. In many cases, we still have no idea whether the combinations we are using will be effective. Of course, the efficacy of the combination depends not only on the active constituents of each of the component herbs, but also on constituents which may not be active but may nevertheless interfere with the active constituents of other herbs. If we combine, for instance, herbs containing alkaloids with those containing a high level of tannins, this may slow down the absorption of the active alkaloids or sometimes inactivate the alkaloids altogether. Conversely, herbs with active constituents that are quickly absorbed can be deliberately combined with herbs rich in tannins in order to slow the absorption of the active ingredient.

A number of herbs have more than one action. A common approach in herbal medicine is to combine a number of herbs with an affinity for a particular system or organ, in order to approach the problem from several directions – a kind of blunderbuss effect. Unfortunately the efficacy of such combinations is often compromised owing to the inactivation of one herb by another: for example, prescriptions given to patients with circulatory problems often contain both *Valeriana officinalis*, a relaxant and sedative and *Zanthoxylum* spp., an arterial stimulant whose separate actions tend to cancel each other out. The resulting effect, therefore, is much less than if the two medicines were given separately, say *Zanthoxylum* in the morning and *Valeriana officinalis* in the afternoon.

In summary, combinations should only be made between herbs which either have similar actions – such as sedatives and relaxants – or which are thought to work on one and the same system of the body, and even then the possibility of one constituent rendering another inactive must be borne in mind. For example, prescriptions for the cardiovascular system often contain both hawthorn (*Crataegus* spp.) and cramp bark (*Viburnum opulus* L.). Observing this mixture over a number of days, one will see that a substantial amount of precipitation builds up in the bottle. One is forced to conclude that some hawthorn constituents are precipitated by the tannins in the cramp bark. This combination, therefore, should not be made and the herbs should be given separately. On the other hand, *Viburnum opulus* can be safely combined with chamomile (*Matricaria recutita* L.) or *Valeriana officinalis*, as can *Crataegus* spp. with lily of the valley (*Convallaria majus* L.).

Mono or polypharmacy

Some 30 to 50 years ago there was a strong tendency towards polypharmacy in herbal medicine: at that time an average prescription might contain 20 herbs or more. Given the current state of knowledge about the multiple constituents of herbs, we must admit the possibility that combining 10 or 15 herbs will lead to a substantial interaction between the different constituents. It is often impossible to calculate the end-result of mixing several active constituents in the same bottle. It has therefore become common practice over the last decade to reduce the number of herbs used in a prescription to the bare minimum. The licensing authorities now even demand, with very few exceptions, that a product requiring a licence contain no more than two or three herbs.

In cases where treatment requires more than four or five herbs the prescription can be broken down into two or more components.

There are other reasons why we should not use too many herbs in one prescription. It is now known that many processes in the body are not single simple actions but, rather, combinations of different mechanisms which work together, sometimes in tandem, sometimes in sequence, to obtain the desired result. For instance, expectoration can be achieved by the reflex action of saponins on the gut mucosa, by the direct action on the respiratory mucosa of certain volatile oils, or by stimulation of the 'ciliary escalator' of the URT. Some herbs have a specific mode of action and need to be given at a certain concentration. It is better to use one herb in sufficient quantity than two or three in quantities insufficient to trigger the desired mechanism.

The process of diuresis, again, can be due to several mechanisms: (a) an increased glomerular filtration rate; (b) increased osmotic pressure of the fluid in the tubules; or (c) suppression of reabsorption of Na+ and CI- ions by the tubules. Each process can be activated by different herbs.

Dandelion (*Taraxacum officinale* Spp.) leaf, for example, is active in suppressing the reabsorption of Na+ and CI- ions in the tubular fluid (saluretic). To obtain a substantial increase in diuresis, however, a considerable amount of dandelion leaf is required – at least 1-2 ml dandelion leaf FE/kg body weight/day. The same principle is true for the other mechanisms as well; for example the rate of diuresis due to osmosis depends on the amount of ions, salts, or sugars dissolved. In practical terms, a prescription directed towards increased diuresis, say in a case of hypertension and oedema, that aims for a blunderbuss effect by including some five to ten diuretics may result in no diuretic action at all as there is no single diuretic present at a sufficiently high dose.

Splitting up the prescription

Regrettably few practitioners use the technique of breaking up a prescription into at least two components, and sometimes three or more, to suit the patient. With this method the make-up of the components, and the timing of the administration, can be determined according to the considerations discussed above: the time factor, whether the medicine is best taken before or after meals, unsuitable combinations, and so on.

For example, our prescription could contain a herb acting on the nervous system, to be taken first thing in the morning as a single dose; then a mixture to be taken before breakfast and lunch, containing both a trophorestorative for the kidney and echinacea, whose active sugar components require quick absorption and are unable to withstand an extended period in the stomach; and, finally, a mixture to be taken after meals, containing constituents such as pain-killers and sedatives that would interact with those taken before meals. Echinacea would be given again before the evening meal, and once or twice more before retiring. Sleeping mixtures should be given separately, up to an hour before bedtime. Putting all these components in one and the same bottle would drastically reduce the actions of the herbs and their remedial value for the patient.

Standardisation and quality control

Contrary to what many people believe, a tincture is not just any alcoholic extract of a medicinal plant. An official tincture, as defined by the *British Pharmacopoeia* or *British Pharmaceutical Codex*, is an alcoholic plant extract obtained by the process of maceration or percolation and using a defined amount of herb (usually dried) extracted with a specific amount of an alcohol/water mixture of a specific strength.

Over the years we have found that preparations differ quite considerably in quality and strength from batch to batch and also between the different producers of tinctures. It is of course of the utmost importance in herbal medicine, especially as regards tinctures, that the preparations should always be of a known strength, since it is now clear that certain herbs only have an effect if given in a sufficient dose, usually calculated from one of the active constituents. Only if the strength of the tincture is known for example, if we know how much of the active constituent is present per ml of tincture, can we prescribe with confidence.

Ideally, we should aim for harmonization in the future, so that herbal medicines in general are of the same strength from whatever source they are obtained. An alternative solution would be to state on the label the strength, expressed in milligrams or grams, of the active constituent per unit of tincture. Strict quality control should be implemented, starting with the crude drug for example, the dried or fresh herb. It is imperative that practitioners understand that standardization and quality control are of the utmost importance, and that they should be applied with the same rigour in the preparation of alternative medicines as they are in that of orthodox pharmaceuticals.

Herbal Philosophy

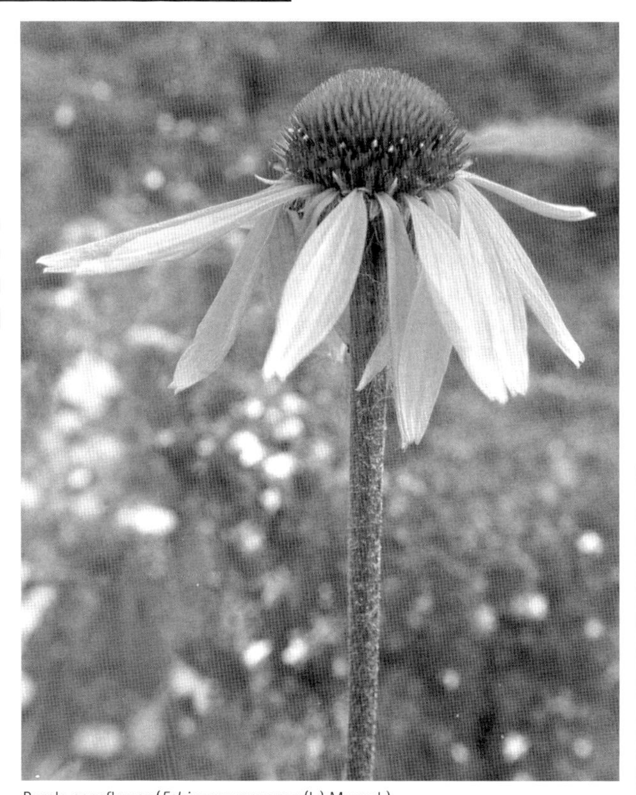

Purple coneflower (*Echinacea purpurea* (L.) Moench)

A brief introduction to the Hippocratic tract 'On Airs, Waters, and Places' for Western herbalists

Robyn James

The Hippocratic Corpus is one of the most significant collections of texts for those studying the history of Western medicine. Many overt influences of the Corpus persist in herbal medicine today, from the swearing of the Hippocratic oath to the separation of acute from chronic diseases, and so it is also likely that more subtle assumptions derived from these texts pervade our culture as Western herbalists. A familiarity with their original sources could help in evaluating the importance of such systems and beliefs within our modern practices.

The Hippocratic Corpus

The collection as a whole consists of around 60 treatises traditionally attributed to the great physician Hippocrates, c. 460–c377 BCE (Nutton 2004). Although it is certainly possible that some of the tracts may have been written by Hippocrates himself, none can now be attributed to him with any certainty, and today the whole work is considered to have many different authors. Indeed, some of the tracts present completely contradictory viewpoints, and a few clearly base their doctrines on those taught at the rival school at Cnidus rather than the Hippocratic school in Cos (Lloyd 1978). The tracts are mostly dated at between 430 and 330 BCE and it is probable that they were first compiled by scholars working at Alexandria at around the third century BCE (Nutton 2004). However, there is some evidence of later additions, including some that were clearly composed much later than 330 BCE (Lloyd 1978).

The tracts vary in their nature and purpose, with some being obviously intended for a general, including lay, audience; others specifically address medical students or physicians. Some are scraps or case notes; some carefully composed lectures; others are practical manuals. Many attempts have been made to identify individual authors of individual tracts, but the evidence available is poor and conflicting, and none can be positively identified.

On Airs, Waters, and Places

On Airs, Waters, and Places, for which English translations can be found online (Stevenson 1994), is a short tract of less than 10,000 words split into 24 parts, and is perhaps one of the easiest and most appealing Hippocratic texts for a Western herbalist to begin with. In fact, it was a key text for Western physicians until the mid-nineteenth century, being regularly republished with new commentaries for the physician (Miller 1962). It is a core treatise of the collection, being almost certainly from Cos, and was one of the few still considered to be the personal work of Hippocrates right into the late nineteenth century (Jones 1868).

It appears to have been composed as advice for itinerant physicians, to give them a guide to the diseases they are likely to encounter in different places at different times of year. Such travelling physicians would have needed to rapidly establish their skills in order to make a living, as there were no formal professional qualifications that could provide evidence of expertise for a doctor at this time (Lloyd 1970). Despite this practical intention, like all the other texts of the Corpus it is written in the Ionic dialect of Greek even though this was neither the dialect of Cos nor of most of the postulated authors (Nutton 2004). This choice suggests that the writers were educated within the Ionic tradition of learning originally associated with the sixth-century philosophers of Miletus: Thales, Anaximander and Anaximenes. Indeed, like these philosophers, *On Airs, Waters, and Places* provides a broadly rational explanation of the causes of disease, avoiding supernatural explanations wherever possible. 'Each disease has a natural cause and nothing happens without a natural cause' (Part 22).

The influence of Empedocles of Acragas (c. 490–430 BCE) can also be seen in *On Airs, Waters, and Places*. Empedocles developed the idea that all substances were derived from varying proportions of four irreducible elements of primary qualities: cold and dry earth, cold and damp water, hot and damp air and hot and dry fire (Campbell 2014). This fourfold concept is intrinsic to the worldview presented in *On Airs, Waters, and Places*, which explains natural phenomena in the same fourfold terms of a universe of four primary qualities and four elements. Here the approach is extended to groupings of the north and south, east and west winds; the spring and autumn, summer and winter; cold and hot, dry and moist climates. In the same way as for earth, air, fire and water, each of these groups is characterised as two complementary pairs of opposites, with each pole being associated with qualities that would be reflected in the people exposed to them.

So, according to *On Airs, Waters, and Places*, cities facing south, that is sheltered from the north and therefore exposed to hot winds will have inhabitants 'of a humid and pituitous constitution' subject to disorders of heat such as dysentery and chronic fevers in winter. Cities facing north, exposed to cold winds, will have hardy inhabitants prone to cold, dry disorders such as constipations. Cities facing east are the healthiest as such a situation 'resembles the spring', and have few diseases. As a native of such a fortunately placed city, I am utterly convinced by the claim that the local populace would be 'well coloured and blooming ... and in temper and intellect are superior.' This certainly has the ring of truth to me! By contrast, those cities facing west are subject to dampness (think of Manchester) and bear 'a great resemblance to autumn'. This is the most unhealthy of all. The residents are 'pale and enfeebled'.

Microcosm of the macrocosm

It can also be seen from this fourfold approach that the author believes the same laws that govern natural processes in the larger world can be seen within man as 'a microcosm of the macrocosm'. This idea, that the structure of man parallels and corresponds to the structure of the universe, is usually dated to Plato's *Timaeus* of c. 360 BCE. However, it is likely that the concept itself is much older and akin to the astrological premise of a 'sympathy' between the heavenly bodies and earthly life (Wiener 1973). In *On Airs, Waters, and Places*, this idea is explicitly stated in a poetic description at the end of Part 14 which says 'the nature of some [men] is like to a country covered with trees and well watered; of some, to a thin soil deficient in water; of others, to fenny and marshy places; and of some again, to a plain of bare and parched land.' Note that this is yet another example of the use of two complementary pairs of opposites.

The qualities present in the external universe are reflected in the 'humours' (body fluids) that relate to them in making up the internal universe of the body. In line with its characterisation of the universe in terms of complementary pairs of opposites, *On Airs, Waters, and Places* refers to four humours: phlegm, bile, blood and melancholy, making the implicit assumption that health is the harmonious (although not necessarily equal) mixture of the four. However, a belief in a total of four humours is by no means universal in the whole Hippocratic Corpus. Even in the other texts that do refer to four, sometimes water is substituted for melancholy (Pitman 2006).

As the balance of the humours reflects the qualities present in the external environment, they will naturally vary with the locale and seasons. Part 10 describes how seasons that were excessively hot or cold, dry or damp for the time of year would disturb this cyclical variation and cause disease via excess of the corresponding humours. Although this description is largely based on doctrine rather than observation, the writer also accurately describes malaria and the circumstances that lead to it becoming epidemic, which suggests both familiarity with real medical practice and some acceptance of the value of empiricism (Porter 1999).

In Part 11, *On Airs, Waters, and Places* suggests that changes of the seasons, solstices, equinoxes and the dates when significant stars rise (used to date the starts and ends of seasons) are inauspicious times when disease is particularly likely to become dangerous and surgery must be avoided. Although no explanation is given in this tract, other Hippocratic texts suggest that this belief was made rational by associating melancholy with change and hence with these critical dates, although the belief itself probably pre-dates such theory (Pitman 2006). Excess of any humour could cause disease, but excess of melancholy appears to be particularly dangerous.

Parts 12 to 24, which may actually have once been a separate essay (Miller 1962), describe the relationship of climatic and geographic factors with national characteristics of various countries in Asia, northern Africa and Europe. There are enticing descriptions of Macrocephali with their elongated heads; the Sauromatae (Amazons) with their right breasts removed; and wagon-dwelling Scythians, amongst others. As in Parts 1–11, the author reports that the qualities associated with the natural phenomena in the external environment will be reflected in the people. For example, those from mountainous rugged lands display qualities of cold, such as a warlike disposition. Asians, from the spring-like East, are described as mild in temperament. However, in the second part, the four-fold arrangement becomes less important than the impact on people of change in the macrocosm – in this case changeability of climate. The Asian mildness is attributed more to the lack of variation in their climate rather than to their location in the East. This suggests that this second part of the tract may indeed be a separate work from the first, and has likely been influenced more by the philosopher Heraclitus who emphasised the importance of change in the world (Lloyd 1970).

The legacy

Twenty-first century Western medical herbalism embraces a broad spectrum of approaches. It is reassuring to see that this has such a long history – even the Hippocratic collection displays some utterly contradictory views. Perhaps such diversity should be considered to be a valuable and intrinsic part of our philosophy. The ability to draw ideas from different systems widens the range of therapeutic possibilities that we can offer to our patients.

The influence of the four-fold arrangement of the microcosm and macrocosm is rather subtle but similar four-fold systems continued to structure Western systems of healthcare for centuries after Hippocrates. For example, the parallels should be obvious for any herbalists taught the physiomedical system of classifying bodily functions as stimulated/sedated and contracted/relaxed (Priest and Priest 1983). Similar ideas can be seen in the Jungian concepts that contrast the conscious and unconscious mind: 'life is born only of the spark of opposites' (Jung 1967). By contrast, Eastern traditional medical systems are generally structured around concepts that come in threes, such as the Ayurvedic doshas; or in fives, such as the Chinese elements.

Furthermore, while Western herbalists today rarely have a widely peripatetic practice, the detail of how *On Airs, Waters, and Places* posits the health of the individual within the wider context of their location is highly thought provoking. We might argue with the details and the reasons given in the text, but the physical environment inevitably shapes the life forms that inhabit it. Our focus as medical herbalists tends to be on the individual in front of us, and so there is always a risk that the wider context could be lost. This text reminds us that the health of the individual is indivisible from the health of the community and ecosystem.

Another striking element of the text is the use of metaphor. As well as being part of the ecosystem, diseases and people are likened to them. Such use of metaphor is now all too rare in Western medicine, which tends to shun subjective descriptions. However, similar comparisons could certainly help to illustrate any discussion of the complex ecosystems of micro-organisms now known to inhabit our bodies.

The Hippocratic texts are one of the foundations on which Western herbal medicine has been built. Revisiting these texts, opening up the ways in which they have influenced our practice nowadays, is a way to ground our practice within our own cultural heritage. This allows us to reassess the importance of some persistent beliefs and practices, whilst also reminding us of alternative ways of thinking about health and disease. The philosophical framework of Western herbal medicine is eclectic, drawing from history as well as from modern research, and so these texts deserve to be given new attention.

References

Campbell, G. 2014. *Empedocles.* [online] *The internet encyclopedia of philosophy.* Available from http://www.iep.utm.edu/empedocl/ [Accessed 7 June 2014].

Jones, W.H.S. 1868. Introduction in *Hippocrates collected works Vol 1.* Trans Jones , W.H.S. Cambridge MA: Harvard University Press, 1868.

Jung, C.G. 1967. Two essays on analytical psychology. In: Jung, C.G. *Collected works of C.G. Jung,* Volume 7. Princeton, N.J.: Princeton University Press.

Lloyd, G.E.R. 1970. *Early Greek science: Thales to Aristotle.* London: Chatto & Windus.

Lloyd, G.E.R. ed. (1978) *Hippocratic writings.* Harmondsworth: Penguin.

Miller, G. 1962. 'Airs, Waters, and Places' in history. *Journal of the history of medicine and allied sciences,* 17(1) 129–40.

Nutton, V. 2004. *Ancient medicine.* Abingdon: Routledge.

Pitman, V. 2006. *The nature of the whole: holism in Ancient Greek and Indian medicine.* Delhi: Motilal Banarsidass Ltd.

Porter, R. 1999. *The greatest benefit to mankind: a medical history of humanity from antiquity to the present.* London: Fontana Press.

Priest, A.W. and Priest L.R. 2000. *Herbal medication: a clinical and dispensary handbook.* Saffron Walden: The C.W. Daniel Company Ltd.

Stevenson, D. C. 1994. *The internet classics archive.* [online] Massachusetts: Massachusetts Institute of Technology. Available from http://classics.mit.edu/ [Accessed 7 June 2014]

Wiener, Philip P. ed. 1973. *Dictionary of the history of ideas.* [online] New York: Charles Scribner's Sons. Available from http://xtf.lib.virginia.edu/xtf/view?docId=DicHist/uvaBook/tei/DicHist3.xml;chunk.id=dv3-16;toc.depth=1;toc.id=dv3-16;brand=default [Accessed 8 May 2011].

Further reading

Barker, J. 2007. *History, philosophy and medicine: phytotherapy in context.* Kent: Winter Press.

Johnson, J.W. 1960. Of differing ages and climes. *Journal of the history of ideas*, 21 465–80.

Longrigg, J. 1993. *Greek rational medicine.* London: Routledge.

Some thoughts on a common philosophical perspective

Andrew Chevallier

Introduction

While traditional Chinese medicine (TCM) and Ayurveda are traditional medicine systems that for the most part have retained a continuity in their perspectives on health, illness and therapeutics over the centuries, Western herbal medicine has a more fractured history. One hundred and fifty years on from the founding of the National Institute of Medical Herbalists (NIMH), it is interesting to ask whether there are ideas and perspectives on health and therapeutics – that were commonly shared by medical herbalists in 1864 – that are still extant today. My guess would be not that many. But, if few of the philosophical perspectives of 1864 have survived through to 2014, what do we believe in today?

Below, I have listed a number of short paragraphs that I think – to a greater or lesser degree – summarise some of the core beliefs or perspectives that underpin our practice as medical herbalists in 2014. These paragraphs are *not* intended to be read as being *true*. It is up to the reader to agree or disagree with these statements, and to decide to what degree they are true or false. The aim is to stimulate some thought. These paragraphs represent a small and very incomplete beginning.

Some ideas that underpin Western herbal medicine

1. Health and illness

Prevention is better than cure.

Illness results from disequilibrium or disharmony within the individual, which may manifest as physiological, emotional or mental disturbance, ie, disturbed homeostasis (though homeostasis does not necessarily imply health).

The 'terrain', ie, the internal physiological environment (itself shaped by neuro-endocrine/emotional influences), is more important in the development of illness than the 'germ' (ie, pathogens); from this it follows that treatment of the individual can be more productive than treatment of the disease, especially in chronic ill health. These two treatment approaches are not mutually exclusive.

Neuro-endocrine function represents the highest level of physiological organisation and activity, though this function is itself dependent on effective systemic and organic function – especially immune, cardiovascular, digestive and eliminatory.

Ill health is rarely unifactorial and is usually multifactorial in origin – the more chronic the ill health, the more this is liable to be the case.

Signs and symptoms of illness can be understood as expressions or communications of disorder. The body can be seen as an intelligent, organised system.

Health is a dynamic state, in which the individual's capacity to act on, or adapt to, the challenges of external forces (from the cellular level upwards) is close to the optimum; by and large, health only occurs when the internal environment of the body is in accord with the external environment.

2. Treatment

"First the word, then the herb, lastly the knife", (Asclepius c. 1200 BCE, quoted in Weiss 1988): education/talking therapy comes before medication, medication comes before surgery.

"If the patient can be treated through diet alone, he should not be treated with medicines. If (not) ... choose medicines that are nourishing & foods that have medicinal properties. Only if these are insufficient should one use stronger medicines" (Maimonides, on the Art of Healing, quoted in Greenbaum 1995).

Herbal medicine exerts a positive, supportive influence on the body. This can be used to maintain or enhance good health, to treat illness and to aid recovery.

Recovery from illness is due, in the last instance, to the self-healing processes of the body/mind/spirit of the individual; medication and remedial treatment of any kind act to either support or hinder this process.

3. The plants

Medicinal plants span the continuum that runs from food to medicine to poison. As a generalisation, plants can act as food, medicine or poison depending on the dosage used; in any given situation, the aim is to use the lowest effective dosage and the best tolerated herbs for the patient concerned.

Herbal extracts that are close to their natural state (and level of dilution) are more likely to be well tolerated than concentrated extracts.

Medicinal plants and simple extracts are particularly well-suited to supporting self-healing processes, promoting effective digestion, absorption, metabolism and elimination, and mitigating the effects of acute or chronic stress.

The dilute dosage and synergistic interaction of the complex of constituents within medicinal plants means that they tend to support rather than override normal physiological function and self-healing processes; combinations of different medicinal plants extend this idea of synergistic activity further, different plants and constituents reinforcing the activity of other plants and constituents.

4. The therapeutic relationship

Particular lifestyles, including home and working environments and exposure to pollutants, level and type of exercise, diet and nutrition, and mental, emotional and spiritual outlook, predispose to specific types of illness; advice on lifestyle that minimises risks of developing ill health and promotes self-healing is an integral part of medical herbalism.

Therapeutic strategies vary depending on the severity and chronicity of the ill health and the loss of vital reserves involved; the vital reserve or force is that part of the body/mind/spirit that actively maintains health, homeostatic function and mental and emotional equilibrium; assessment of the state of the vital or energetic force of the patient is often the starting point when reviewing the therapeutic opportunities available; traditional strategies that are adopted include stimulating/sedating, heating/cooling, toning/relaxing, drying/moistening.

The development of a caring and trusting relationship between patient and practitioner lies at the heart of herbal practice; clear, effective communication with patients and the encouragement of a positive attitude to health and recovery are essential elements in the therapeutic relationship and themselves aid the healing process.

Herbal practice involves working intelligently with natural complexity and variability, as found in both individual patients and medicinal plants; as such, empirical knowledge – derived from practical experience, may often be as or more relevant in guiding decision making than rational knowledge – derived from scientific experimentation.

This distinction between empirical and rational knowledge parallels the distinction found between traditional (experiential) and scientific (experimental) knowledge.

The practice of contemporary medical herbalism requires practitioners to have a structured, scientific knowledge base that encompasses the medical, pharmaceutical and botanical sciences. With this scientific base in place, practitioners are able to derive experiential knowledge based on their practical experience of treating patients. As with many professions and crafts, developed experiential knowledge manifests as intuition. This takes time.

'The Life so short, the Craft so long to learn', Hippocrates' most famous maxim, states this (above) idea more elegantly.

5. And ...

An energetic or vibrational perspective of health and illness and of medicinal plant activity, which as yet has little scientific validation, is frequently the best way of explaining or understanding traditional or experiential herbal knowledge.

Conclusion

We will have a healthy future only in so far as we are willing to make a stand on *our* experience and beliefs, and *our* ability to select and develop the intellectual 'tools' of our craft.

References

Greenbaum A., 1995. *The wings of the sun: traditional Jewish healing in theory and practice.* Jerusalem: Breslov Research Institute.

Weiss R.F., 1988. *Herbal medicine.* Stuttgart; Thieme Publishing Group.

Further reading

Chevallier, A., 1993. *Herbal first aid: a guide to home use.* Rochester: Amberwood Publishing.

Chevallier, A., 1996/2001. *Encyclopedia of herbal medicine.* London: Dorling Kindersley Publishing.

Chevallier, A., 1998. *Phytotherapy: 50 Vital herbs.* Rochester: Amberwood Publishing.

Chevallier, A., 2001. *Herbal medicine for the menopause.* Rochester: Amberwood Publishing.

Chevallier, A., 2007. *Herbal remedies.* London: Dorling Kindersley Publishing.

Coffin A.I., 1866. *Coffin's botanic guide to health.* London: Friendly Botanic Society of Britain.

Swinburne C.R., 1905/1997. *Nature's healing agents.* Philadelphia: Dorrance.

Font Quer P., 1961/1981. *Plantas medicinales: el dioscorides renovado.* Barcelona: Penninsula.

Priest, A.W., and Priest, L.R., 1982. *Herbal medication.* Romford: L.N. Fowler.

Valnet J., 1982. *The practice of aromatherapy.* London: C.W. Daniel.

Pietroni P.C., 1987. *The meaning of illness – holism dissected.* Available from: http://www.ncbi.nlm.nih.gov/pmc/articles/PMC1290855/?page=1.

Complexity and herbal practice

Peter Conway

As a living tradition the practice of herbal medicine modulates and adapts in response to changes in the cultural context in which it operates. Some of the forces catalysing and shaping such change can also enable us to view herbal practice in new ways, opening new potentials for therapeutic interventions and the explanation/justification of such. As we take stock of the herbal present and speculate on herbal futures it may be helpful to consider matters through the scrying lens of complexity theory – an evolving model that is profoundly affecting our understanding of science, society and medicine – and one which, I believe, can validate, illuminate and potentiate herbal practice.

The development of conventional medical science has been characterised by reductionism. The narrow application of reductionism when applied to medicinal plants leads to a focus on key active phytochemical constituents that risks losing sight of, or even misrepresenting, the activity of the whole plant. When applied to medical conditions, this leads to a focus on cellular and other micro-processes that tend to lose sight of the whole person. Thus reductionism is an approach that veers to accumulating fine detail whilst shedding a broader perspective.

Reductionism is nothing new. Paracelsus (1493-1541) said: '...what the eye perceives in herbs or stone or trees is not yet a remedy; the eye sees only the dross. The remedy must be cleansed from the dross, then it is there.' (Griggs 1997). This alchemical dream has been realised in modern pharmacology of course.

Reductionism and holism are not incompatible however – each approach can inform the other. Indeed, when the two are separated from each other the spectrum of understanding has been reduced at both poles. Reductionism set adrift from a holistic perspective tends to abstraction and irrelevance (and even harm); whilst when holism eschews the insights of reductionism it gravitates toward flakiness and incoherence (and inefficacy).

The concept of 'complexity' offers a means of renewing, integrating, and transcending the reductionism–holism polarity. As such it may be a vehicle that can carry us beyond the current conventional-alternative medicine impasse.

The reductionism-holism pairing can be considered as a formulation of the notion of microcosm-macrocosm (to return to alchemy for a moment), where nature is understood to exhibit similar processes or patterns over different scales. For example: an atom has a central nucleus surrounded by orbits of electrons (microcosm), whilst a solar system has a central sun surrounded by orbits of planets (macrocosm). One of the key concepts involved in understanding complexity theory is that of 'fractals'. Fractals describe phenomena that exhibit self-similarity across different scales; e.g. the composition of ferns or lungs, where small segments (for instance terminal bronchioles to use the case of lungs) are composed similarly to larger parts (the main bronchus of the lungs in this example) of the same structure. Benoit Mandelbrot is considered to be the father of fractals and his early paper on this considered the coastline of Britain as a fractal phenomenon (Mandelbrot 1967).

It is worth pausing before proceeding to note Strumia's (2007) observation that much of the language used in connection with the sciences of complexity: 'sound(s) similar, even if not identical, to some (Latin) terms of ancient (Greek and Medieval) philosophy of nature, metaphysics and logic', such as complexity/complexio, chaos/quies, dynamics/motus, self-similarity/similitudo, etc. Complexity can be seen then as an idea with deep roots and many branches – even as a re-engagement with an ancient project. To the extent that it can be portrayed as touching on ancient philosophy and metaphysics, complexity tends to unsettle arch-reductionists when applied to the field of healthcare – the rest of us need not let our curiosity or excitement be dampened.

Above all the reductionist approach is a quest for certainty. The greatest gift of complexity to healthcare may be as a means of living with uncertainty.

Complexity is variously defined amongst authorities but it is important at the outset to state that there is a difference between 'complex' and 'complicated.' Something complicated, such as a computer, is not complex in the way that a living organism is. Camazine *et al.* (2001) define complexity thus:

> *'Complexity and complex systems... generally refer to a system of interacting units that displays global properties not present at the lower level. These systems may show diverse responses that are often sensitively dependent on both the initial state of the system and nonlinear interactions among its components. Since these nonlinear interactions involve amplification or cooperativity, complex behaviours may emerge even though the system components may be similar and follow simple rules.'*

Mitchell (2009) considers the study of complex systems to be:

> *'...an interdisciplinary field of research that seeks to explain how large numbers of relatively simple entities organize themselves, without the benefit of any central controller, into a collective whole that creates patterns, uses information, and, in some cases, evolves and learns. The word complex comes from the Latin root plectere: to weave, entwine. In complex systems, many simple parts are irreducibly entwined, and the field of complexity is itself an entwining of many different fields.'*

Complex systems include insect colonies, immune systems, brains, economies, ecosystems, and the weather.

In a classic early paper Simon (1962) argues that complex systems are essentially hierarchical: 'the complex system being composed of subsystems that, in turn, have their own subsystems, and so on.' He also speculates on the relationship between complexity and simplicity: 'we could expect complex systems to be hierarchies in a world in which complexity had to evolve from simplicity.' A core idea in complexity remains that relatively simple basic interactions between core components generate complexity.

Characteristics of complex systems include:

- sensitivity to initial conditions
- attractors
- nonlinearity

- self-organisation
- emergent properties

Very brief comments on these follow, but beware – each of the characteristics just listed are, well, complex – and contested – the following provides an orientation for further exploration only (there is little that is truly definitive at this stage in the development of complexity science).

Sensitivity to initial conditions:

Complex systems give rise to emergent properties that are dependent on – but not always predictable by knowledge of – the initial conditions of the system. Chaotic systems are especially sensitive to initial conditions such that even very small variations in starting parameters can lead to widely diverging outcomes.

So we need to talk about chaos for a second...

'Chaos' is a term used to describe dynamical systems with sensitive dependence on initial conditions. It can be considered as a phenomenon that is part of complexity theory. Although chaotic systems are unpredictable at the detailed level they are not lacking in mathematical order (such as period-doubling and Feigenbaum's constant) – which means that 'higher-level' aspects of chaos can be predictable (i.e. certain general patterns of behaviour emerge).

Which brings us to the notion of the 'edge of chaos'...

The edge of chaos is variously described but may be considered with reference to the changing states of water. We can see ice as fixed order and water as complex (disordered), whereas the gaseous vapour state of water is chaotic (highly disordered). The transitions from ice to water and from water to gas are 'phase transitions.' The territory around the transition from water to gas – from a disordered to a highly disordered state – is the edge of chaos.

Attractors

One of the best-known examples of mathematical chaos is the Lorenz attractor – better known as the butterfly attractor (when Lorenz's attractor is plotted out visually it looks somewhat like a pair of butterfly's wings). In 1959 Edward Lorenz was studying weather patterns using non-linear equations running on the basic computer systems of the time

– his data outputs were simple lists of numbers. He found that slight variations in data input could lead to large divergences in output. His serendipitous discovery involved running sequences from 0.506 and 0.506127 and finding that the 'model was so sensitive to initial conditions that the difference, one quarter of one tenth of 1 per cent, made the two runs diverge completely from one another after a short time' (Gribbin 2005). In 1972 Lorenz published a playfully titled paper: 'Does the flap of a butterfly's wings in Brazil set off a tornado in Texas?' which has led to the popular notion of the 'butterfly effect.'

As Gribbin (2005) puts it, Lorenz's example suggested that 'a small nudge from outside may be all that it takes to shift a system from a trajectory.'

Attractors are final behaviours that may be attained from a set of initial conditions – the initial conditions are said to be 'attracted to' these eventual behaviours, which are of different types including: 'fixed point'; 'oscillatory'; and 'chaotic'. Chaotic attractors are sometimes termed 'strange attractors'.

Nonlinearity:

Complex systems exhibit nonlinearity – a property that enables the characteristic of sensitivity to initial conditions and leads to chaotic outcomes. Linear systems can be appreciated by understanding the component parts – in nonlinear systems outcomes are not necessarily equal to the sum of the parts.

Self-organisation:

> *'Self-organisation is a process in which pattern at the global level of a system emerges solely from numerous interactions among the lower-level components of the system. Moreover, the rules specifying interactions among the system's components are executed using only local information, without reference to the global pattern... interactions among system components can be surprisingly simple, even when extremely sophisticated patterns are built, such as the labyrinthine nest of termites, the spatial patterns of army ant raids, and the coordinated movements of fish in a school... A striking feature of self-organized systems is the occurrence of a bifurcation – a sudden transition from one pattern to another following even a small change in a parameter of the system. One speaks of 'tuning'*

a parameter in the system to invoke the onset of a different pattern... By making small adjustments in such parameters, one can induce large changes in the state of the system, since the system may now be on a trajectory that flows to a quite different attractor. Most self-organized systems have many tunable parameters' (Camazine *et al.* 2001).

Emergent properties

These are phenomena that arise out of complex systems and which are not predictable from knowledge of the initial conditions. Both health and illness/disease may be considered as emergent properties. Discussion of how complex systems actually work is beyond the scope of this paper but methods include:

- signalling
- feedback
- rules
- stigmergy (subsequent action influenced by action previously taken)
- cues
- cooperation
- amplification

All of these means of producing complexity operate within plants and people.

As a point of departure leading into the consideration of complexity in health and illness/disease let us consider homoeostasis:

Claude Bernard (1813-1878) famously stated that 'La fixité du milieu interieur est la condition de la vie libre.' Walter Cannon (1871-1945) later coined the term homoeostasis. In his book *The Wisdom of the Body* (1932), Cannon describes homoeostasis as 'the coordinated physiological reactions which maintain most of the steady states in the body.' The notion that normality or health are equated with narrowly fixed stable physiological parameters has stuck but contemporary physiologist Ary Goldberger is one of those who challenges this view:

'Physiologic systems in health and disease display an extraordinary range of temporal behaviours and structural patterns that defy understanding based on linear constructs, reductionist strategies, and classical homeostasis. Application of concepts and

> *computational tools derived from... complex systems, including nonlinear dynamics, fractals and chaos theory, is having an increasing impact on biology and medicine.'* (Goldberger 2006).

And again:

> *'According to classical concepts of physiologic control, healthy systems are self-regulated to reduce variability and maintain physiologic constancy. Contrary to the predictions of homeostasis, however, the output of a wide variety of systems, such as the normal human heartbeat, fluctuates in a complex manner, even under resting conditions'* (Goldberger 2002).

Lloyd *et al.* (2001) have suggested 'homeodynamic' as a term that more accurately captures the nature of healthy physiological functioning:

> *'...biological systems are homeodynamic because of their ability to dynamically self-organise at bifurcation points of their behaviour where they lose stability. Consequently, they exhibit diverse behaviour; in addition to monotonic stationery states, living systems display complex behaviour with all its emergent characteristics... It is dynamic organisation under homeodynamic conditions that make possible the organised complexity of life.'*

The physiologist Bruce McEwen has developed the concept of 'allostasis' (maintaining stability through change) to complement a revised notion of homoeostasis. In McEwen's model homoeostasis refers to those physiological systems that are essential for life and which must be kept within strict parameters (such as pH, body temperature, glucose levels and oxygen tension), whereas allostasis refers to physiological systems (such as hormones and cytokines) that maintain those essential functions 'as environment and life history stages change' (McEwen and Wingfield 2003). Mediators of allostasis (such as glucocorticoids) act to 'integrate physiology and associated behaviours in response to changing environments and challenges'. The allostatic state in an individual can be quantified in terms of 'allostatic load' or, in extremis 'allostatic overload'.

Psychoneuroimmunology (PNI) is developing as an integrated systems approach to physiology that offers a means of appreciating the human organism as a complex system. PNI explores the links between the psyche (meaning – thoughts, emotions, beliefs, behaviours) and the three major control systems of the body: the nervous, immune and endocrine systems. Psychological factors have biochemical consequences and these are traced by PNI. For a sound introduction to the field see Wisneski and Anderson (2005).

The new physiological views of the body reveal it as highly complex, integrated and dynamic. Complexity confers robustness and resilience – especially in the face of change. In fact health might be defined as the ability to cope with change. Whilst certain physiological parameters must be kept within a narrow range others are capable of a wide range of activity. Some authorities now consider that a lack of complexity, or 'too much order', is associated with ill health. Martinez-Lavin, *et al.* (2008), report the finding of decreased heart rate variability and monotonous circadian rhythm patterns in patients with fibromyalgia. They conclude that: 'These anomalies can be interpreted as a 'decomplexification' of the autonomic nervous system'. Burton *et al.* (2009) applied complexity science methods (the type of nonlinear dynamic analysis of physiological data that Ary Goldberger does) to investigate chronic fatigue syndrome and they found 'evidence of reduced complexity of activity patterns'.

'Decomplexification' – 'reduced complexity' – these appear to be crucial characteristics of many medical conditions – especially in chronic illnesses.

Herbs and human beings are complex systems, sharing many commonalities beginning at the cellular level. The crucial difference between conventional drugs and herbal medicines lies in their level of complexity – drugs are chemically simple whereas herbs are chemically complex. Each type of medicine has its role to play but the place of herbs is likely to be increasingly recognised as the ideas of complexity (very) slowly filter through into medical practice and the limitations of conventional drugs are acknowledged. Hotamisligil (2006) talks of the need to find new types of medicines and speculates on what these might be like:

> *'In searching for new and effective therapeutics, it might be useful to use a systems-chemistry approach to modify integrated outcomes rather than targeting single molecules with the hope that the desired systematic effect might be generated. In other words, it is*

> *likely that creating a 'new homoeostasis' will require the modification of more than one target'.*

Now, where on earth might we find such agents?

Herbal medicine is a means of using plant systems to treat human systems – it is complex medicine. The complex nature of herbs does not mean that the practice of herbal medicine is necessarily complex. Rather the traditional medicine practitioner typically stands in awe of the mystery of nature, content to modulate systems activity and modify emergent properties by e.g. 'moving the blood' or 'draining heat'. As greater knowledge of phytochemistry has been gained alongside more detailed information regarding the physiological effects of herbs the potential for integrating traditional and contemporary insights into herbal practice has arisen. This potential has to date been little realised but complexity theory offers a framework for this task.

Suggestions for ways of considering the activity of herbs in the light of complexity theory:

Simplicity

Global strategies, or those aimed at modulating systems or hierarchies, have broad remedial potential. It is not necessary (though it is desirable) to know in fine physiological detail how herbs are working in order for them to do so. Strategies such as 'nervous trophorestoration' or 'tonifying yin qi' may yield profound effects.

Nudging

Earlier we talked about how chaotic phenomena are sensitive to initial conditions – a situation where even very small changes may lead to widely divergent outcomes. In some instances herbs may provide subtle chemical 'nudges' that are sufficient to significantly alter outcomes.

Pushing

Whilst subtle stimuli have a key role to play in chaotic states they may not be adequate to adapt complex systems in the absence of chaos. Mitchell (2009) reminds us that complex signalling requires a 'sufficient summed strength' to be generated and to cause changes. A push, as it were, is required rather than a nudge. (Investigation of 'nudging and pushing' may throw light on the debate around 'low dose' and 'high dose' prescribing.)

Information

Herbs provide the human organism with chemical information. This information is complex, multiple and varying in degrees of subtlety or strength depending on the particular herb/ combination of herbs/ and dosage. Earlier I cited Mitchell stating that complex systems use information to self-organise and learn. Herbal medicines may contribute to these processes.

Tuning

Herbal information provides ways of tuning physiological parameters (such as those involved in allostasis) and mechanisms – such as signalling, feedback, cues, cooperation and amplification.

Attractors in re-configuring initial conditions

Earlier we said that 'attractors' are final behaviours that may be attained from a set of initial conditions. Herbal treatment (including dietary and lifestyle changes) may be interpreted as a contribution towards re-configuring initial conditions leading to an enhanced eventual outcome. The notion of herbs as attractors is useful since attractors take time to 'pull' activity into final stable forms – particularly in well-established chronic disorders it is necessary to allow time for enhanced patterns of behaviour to emerge.

Working at the edge of chaos

In some instances the cumulative effects of herbal treatment may help to create radical changes in the body. This opportunity exists especially where patients can be located at the edge of chaos where a phase transition between disease and health might be possible.

Self-organisation

Commenting on the approach of the psychologist/neurologist Kurt Goldstein (1878-1965), Oliver Sacks (1995) writes:

> *'The function of the physician, he feels... is to be as sensitive as possible to all the resonances and ramifications of illness in the individual, and so help him to achieve a new organization, an equilibrium... One must lead the sick patient through a period of chaos, gently, until he can re-establish a new organization, construct his world anew'.*

Herbal medicines, and the general herbal approach, may act as stimuli to self-organisation and the restoration of healthy function.

Re-complexification

The problems of 'decomplexification' or 'reduced complexity' were mentioned above. Herbs may offer strategies for re-establishing complexity in the body.

In this short piece I do not want to overlook the broader role of dietary advice and lifestyle modification etc in addition to herbs but space does not allow more than a mention of the importance of these areas. Nor do I want to neglect the healing potential of the consultation so I will close by directing readers to my book on that topic (Conway 2011) from which this final statement is an excerpt:

> *'From the perspective of complexity theory we might describe the phytotherapy consultation process as: the interaction of complex living creatures (human beings), using a complex living system of meaning representation (language), and specific complex sense-making strategies (storytelling and story interpretation) to assess the emergent status of the patient and help facilitate self-organisation, specifically through prescription of complex, systems-level medicines (plant remedies)'.*

References

Burton, C. *et al.*, 2009. Reduced complexity of activity patterns in patients with chronic fatigue syndrome: a case control study. *BioPsychoSocial Medicine*, 3, 7.

Camazine, S., *et al.* 2001. *Self-organization in biological systems.* Princeton University Press.

Conway, P., 2011. *The consultation in phytotherapy: the herbal practitioner's approach to the patient.* Elsevier/Churchill-Livingstone.

Goldberger, A.L., *et al.* 2002. Fractal dynamics in physiology: alterations with disease and aging. *PNAS*, 99(1), 2466-72.

Goldberger, A.L., 2006. Complex systems. *Proceedings of the American Thoracic Society*, 3, 467-472.

Gribbin, J., 2005. *Deep simplicity: chaos, complexity and the emergence of life.* Penguin.

Griggs, B., 1997. *Green pharmacy.* Healing Arts Press.

Hotamisligil, G.S., 2006. Inflammation and metabolic disorders. *Nature*, 444(14),860-67.

Lewin, R. 1993. *Complexity: life at the edge of chaos.* Phoenix (Good at conveying the excitement and controversies around complexity – and at mapping the history of its development.)

Lloyd, D.; Aon, M.A and Cortassa, S., 2001. Why homeodynamics, not homeostasis? *The Scientific World Journal*,1,133-145.

Mc Ewen, B.S. and Wingfield, J.C., 2003. The concept of allostasis in biology and medicine. *Hormones and Behaviour*, 43, 2-15.

Mandelbrot, B., 1967. How long is the coast of Britain? Statistical self-similarity and fractional dimension. *Science*, 156, 636-638.

Martinez-Lavin, M., Infante, O. and Lerma, C., 2008. Hypothesis: The chaos and complexity theory may help our understanding of fibromylagia and similar maladies. *Seminars in Arthritis and Rheumatism*, 37(4), 260-264.

Mitchell, M., 2009. *Complexity: a guided tour.* Oxford University Press.

Plsek, P. and Greenhalgh, T., 2001. Complexity science: the challenge of complexity in healthcare. *British Medical Journal*, 323, 625-628.

Plsek, P., Sweeney, K. and Griffiths, F,. 2002. *Complexity and healthcare: an introduction.* Radcliffe.

Sacks, O., 1995. Foreword. *In*: Goldstein, K., *The Organism.* (First published 1954). Zone Books.

Simon, H.A. The architecture of complexity. Proceedings of the American Philosophical Society 1962, 106(6), 467-482.

Strumia, A, 2007. Complexity seems to open a way towards a new Aristotelian-Thomistic ontology. *Acta Biomedica*, 78(1), 32-38.

Sweeney, K., 2006. *Complexity in primary care: understanding its value.* Radcliffe.

Wisneski, L.A. and Anderson, L., 2005. *The scientific basis of integrative medicine.* CRC Press.

Western herbal medicine – back to the future

Jonathan Treasure

Abstract

This article explains the foundations of my work-in-progress concept of Herbalism 3.0. In summary, I divide Western herbal medicine history from the 1st century CE until the end of the 20th CE into two distinct epistemic periods – dubbed Herbalism 1.0 and Herbalism 2.0 (H1.0 & H2.0). I argue that stress lines already visible in H2.0 by the middle of the 20th century, have subsequently matured into seismic faults, which by the year 2000 ushered in a period of crisis (in Khunian terms). This will require a paradigm shift, or a 3.0 iteration of herbal medicine for it to survive, let alone thrive. A dual handicap presents immediate obstacles to developing H3.0. On the one hand, the circumscription of herbalism by 'traditional knowledge' and on the other hand, impoverished scientific support. I would further suggest a third, more serious and subtle challenge which is the adoption of the prevalent mainstream attitude that theory is not practised in the clinic, and consequently can be disregarded, deferred or delegated – since doctoring takes precedence over philosophising when it comes to clinical practice. The net result is that herbalism appears developmentally disabled in relation to the challenges of a future already upon it. This article analyses the epistemic nature of 'herbal medicines' in H1.0 and 2.0, and suggests that a viable H3.0 must draw on the views about the nature or virtues of herbs implied in H1.0.

Introduction

In the opening of a commencement speech titled 'This is water' delivered a few years before his untimely death, David Foster Wallace describes a cameo in which two young fish meet an older fish swimming the other way. As they pass, the older fish nods at them and says "Morning boys! How's the water?" The two young fish swim on by, and a few minutes later one turns to the other and says, "Huh? What is 'water'?" (Foster Wallace 2009). The point of the parable is not so much that we need wise old fish to tell us about the nature of water, but simply that it is often the most obvious and fundamental everyday realities that we find most difficult to talk about.

For western herbalists today, the convenient historic default of not discussing 'the water' is no longer viable. We are confronting challenges that are visibly eroding the viability of our default *modus operandi* and identity, and the sell-by date has long passed. It is quite arguable that herbal medicine has arrived at something of a historic bifurcation point with an increasingly forced choice between two alternative trajectories for the 21st century. The first involves discussing the 'water' – and requires letting go of its 20th century paradigm to meet the challenges of the 21st. The second is the real threat of possible extinction via a combination of sequestration by mainstream biomedicine coupled with fragmentation into various marginalised subcultural cliques and inconsequential factions – a process visibly underway.

The choice of appropriate tools for self-understanding in a field as inherently multi-disciplinarian and heterogeneous as herbalism is not clearly mandated by the specific concerns of its internal content. Nor are herbalists themselves particularly prone to philosophising about their practice. My personal preference is to draw from the toolbox of the history and philosophy of science. Until recently, 'history' in herbal medicine was nearly synonymous with 'tradition' *in sensu* of traditional knowledge. Platitudes of the genre 'combining ancient wisdom with modern science' pervade the marketplace for herbal products, but behind the clichés herbalists have always had a strong sense of the importance of historic continuities in their discipline. Emphasis on the ongoing authority of centuries-old herbals contrasts starkly with the infantile amnesia that typifies modern biomedicine.

Despite this, authoritative historical surveys of western herbalism, with a few exceptions such as Barbara Griggs (Griggs 1981) have been noticeable mostly by their absence. However, several recently published works together make a cogent argument for the emergence of a scholarly approach to the history of herbal medicine by authors clearly literate in both herbalism and history. (Tobyn 2011, Francia and Stobart 2014) My own approach to history is both more pragmatic, philosophical and frankly politicised. Marx famously pointed out that when history repeats itself, the first time is as a tragedy, the second is a farce. Historical self-analysis here is animated above all by the need to learn from and avoid the mistakes of the past. The ulterior motive is not representation but intervention. The study of history conducted as scholastic documentation of how things were done in the past is conservative rather than critical if its implicit programme is 'to stand athwart history yelling 'Stop.''[1]

Like historians, philosophers of science have different motivations and concerns. Here again my preference is hybrid, drawing primarily from the historicism of Kuhn and the anarchy of Feyerabend, but without dispensing altogether with the necessity for internalist analyses of the epistemic content of the science of herbalism itself.[2] This last point is important because adoption of purely sociological or historical approaches to understanding science may be laudable insofar as they emphasise values and ethics as well as cultural relativity and multiperspectivism, but tend to fail in their ability to evaluate internal scientific content; however here I shall rely heavily upon the now 'classical' approach to scientific revolutions developed by Thomas Kuhn. Although familiar to many, a brief review of the main points from *The Structure of Scientific Revolutions* (Kuhn 1962) follows.

Kuhn's scientific revolutions 101

For philosopher of science Thomas Kuhn, a scientific revolution is not simply a shift in the way science views the world, or how and why it performs what experiments. The major scientific revolutions such as heliocentrism, germ theory or general relativity show how new paradigms are associated with profound changes in how we conceive, construct and create our world and thus are world-changing views rather than changing world-views.

In brief, Kuhn posited that historically, science progresses non-linearly with extended periods that he called 'normal science' that were interrupted by periodic crises or revolutions. In the initial period of 'pre-science,' emerging observations and experimental data lead cumulatively to the development of a core disciplinary matrix or 'paradigm' which characterises the period of normal science (business as usual). Over time, anomalous findings may presage the end of business as usual; should those anomalous findings accumulate they can become increasingly 'incommensurable' with the existing paradigm. In this case a period of crisis or 'revolution' ensues, and eventually a new paradigm emerges compatible with the findings that triggered the crisis, and another settled period of normal science follows this 'paradigm shift.' This process is represented below (Fig. 1)

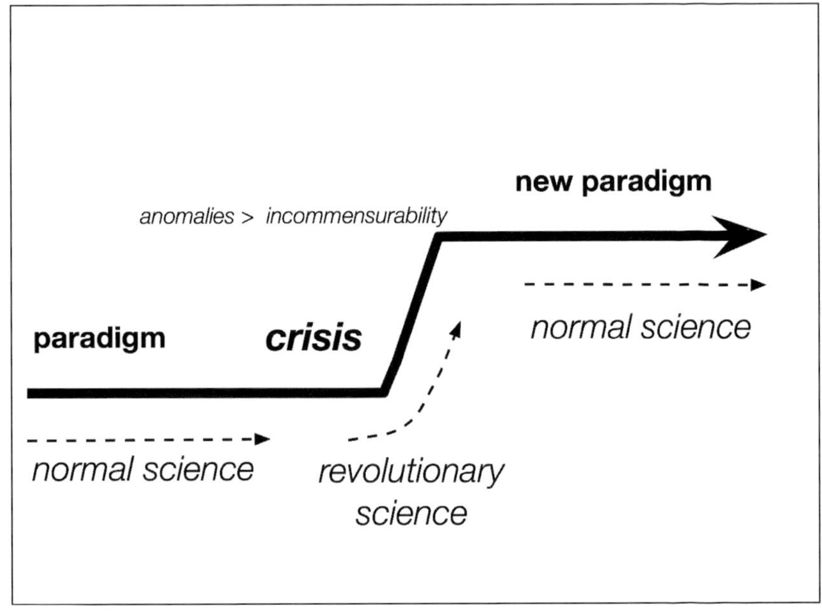

Fig 1. Graphic representation of Kuhnian science

With this framework we can now parse the history of Western herbalism in terms of Khunian paradigms. Doing so involves an inevitable degree of simplification that may risk offending the historicist sensibilities of those more comfortable discussing trees than forests, but our premise is that the forest is ablaze, and maintaining decorum is never a top priority when wildfire fighting. Controversially, my timeline scaling is logarithmic rather than linear, resulting in an unkindly compression of two millennia of herbal medicine into a single chapter. The log scale is also intentionally suggestive of an increasingly urgent need for herbal medicine to recognise the impending Kuhnian crisis, because of the globally accelerated speeds of social, technical and medical developments. For my purposes here, this temporal condensation means Herbalism 1.0 begins with Greco-Roman medicine around the first century CE and Herbalism 2.0 starts at the turn of the 19th Century; this period became

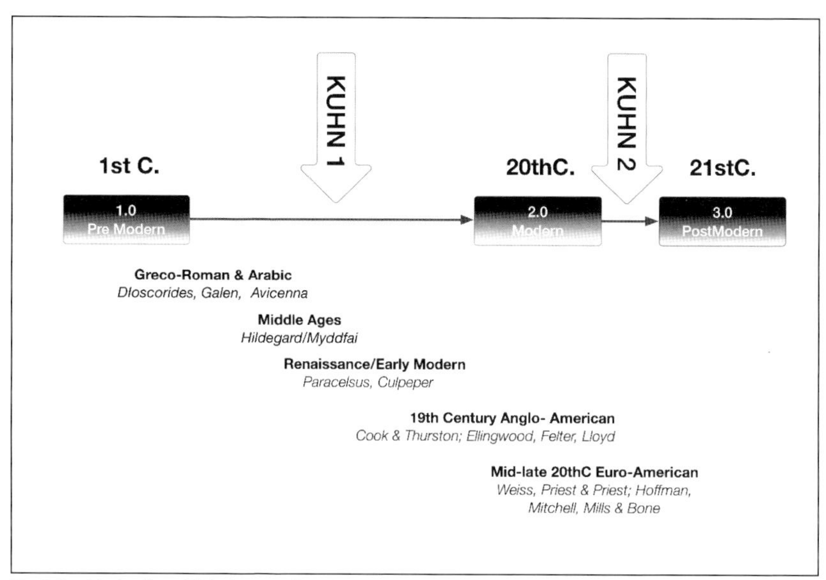

Fig. 2 Graphic timeline of Kuhnian paradigms in western herbal history

'critical' by the turn of the millennium at Y2K, portending a future, but yet to manifest Herbalism 3.0 (Fig. 2).

Herbalism 1.0 – the herbal

Dioscorides is generally regarded as author of the first definitive herbal —an authoritative original knowledge base of botanical remedies, pharmacy and therapeutics (although he included mineral and animal remedies). His *De Materia Medica* is the archetypal expression of Herbalism 1.0 (hereafter H1.0) and of the herbal as a description of the materia medica by the expert practitioner-author.

In terms of medical theory, Dioscorides was more on the empiricist side of the rationalist-empiricist divide that has been identified as a primary animating dialectic of western medical history from the Hippocratic corpus onward, whilst his second-century successor Galen more famously expounded and expanded humoralism – an unreconstructed rationalist in vitalist clothing. However, from the epistemic point of view of herbal medicine, and also of our Kuhnian schema, the medical metaphysics of individual expert-authors are of less significance than the herbal as a scholastic description of their individual expertise and experience with materia medica.

In a way, we can say the herbal is the paradigm. Historic expert-author herbals express a specific conception of the nature of a herbal remedy, of what knowledge of a herb is, and implicitly characterises the nature of the herb. Herbals present the materia medica in terms of the virtues or capacities of each herb. This means that herbal remedies are the kind of things that have the capacity or tendency to behave in different ways depending on who is using them, how, and in what context. Importantly, a herb is not defined by *what it does*, but by what (an expert author-practitioner says) it has *the power to do*. Knowledge of a herb is knowledge of its capacities or virtues, not of its actions. The picture of any herb is painted differently by different herbals and the virtues of a herb can be compiled as a collective aggregate of all its descriptors. The natures of herbs in this sense correspond to their Aristotelian natures, and the accounts of materia medica in herbals owe as much to classical Scholasticism as to empiricism.

It is unclear to what extent the authorial content of the landmark historic herbals of H1.0 is truly primary and original as opposed to derivative, or even plagiaristic. In a later example such as Maud Grieve's *A Modern Herbal* published in 1931, the compilation process is explicit, the sources either acknowledged or at least known; however, in the primary historic herbals (Dioscorides, Gerard *et al.*) this is not necessarily so and is a proper subject for the new wave of herbal historians. However, the existence or extent of 'copycat' descriptions in H1.0 herbals does not undermine the basic features we are focusing on in this text.

I will argue later that a return to the concept of natures is an essential platform for understanding herbs in any Herbalism 3.0. Although the virtues described in H1.0 herbals correspond to natures, Aristotelian natures were always connected to essences. Essences are intrinsically unknowable; indeed the primary achievement of the Scientific Revolution was to banish natures (as unknowable essences) from modern scientific knowledge and methodology as an explanation of the behaviour of things, and replace them by empirically measurable or otherwise knowable indices of what behaviours things exhibit.

In parentheses, from the perspective on history that motivates this text, 17th-century English herbalist Nicholas Culpeper and 16th-century physician/occultist Paracelsus are interesting standouts in the pantheon of H1.0 authors. Each in their own way was uniquely anti-establishment, and each of them eschewed humoralism with its replacement of essences by the rationalist cataloging of energetic qualities, suggesting instead that esoteric methodologies were more appropriate. For Culpeper this was astrology and for Paracelsus alchemy. In the context of their radicalism this could be interpreted as a prescient rejection of the inherent conservatism of humoral rationalism albeit replacing it with esoteric placeholders of alchemy and astrology as a means of 'getting at' essences; in other words acknowledging the shortcomings of humoralism but recognising the need to make the invisible visible. Rendering the essences knowable via motifs of 'as above so below' and alchemical transformation/transcendence has implications for today and the 'making visible' of the capacities or natures of plant medicines and this will be explored in part two of this text in more detail. A less consequential aside is the double irony involved when western herbalists claim historic continuity with humoralism as a vitalist credential against charges that their system is 'inferior' to traditional Asian medical systems due to its lack of comparable energetics of materia medica (or therapeutics).

Herbalism 2.0 – the monograph

The period of crisis in herbal medicine that marked the end of H1.0 spanned the last decades of the 19th century to the first few of the 20th. This transformative time in botanical history was driven by a complex interplay of external socio-political forces that precipitated a Kuhnian crisis period by stressing the already present internal contradictions of the H1.0 paradigm – its inbuilt inability to reparse expertise in materia medica in ways that clearly demarcated both conflicts and compatibilities with the rapidly developing ecosystem of mainstream medicine. The decisive shift was the absolute imperative for herbal medicine to reframe its legitimacy in terms of a medical landscape increasingly dominated by the emerging and bullish pharmaceutical industry in cahoots with a newly confident medical profession whose reductionist thinking underpinned its aggressively expanding socio-economic and clinical hegemony. Only Thurston, in his 1900 *Philosophy of Physiomedicalism*, critically encapsulated the entire dynamics of the historical juncture, and laid the theoretical foundations to meet and transcend its challenges. Still, this was too little too late, and Thurston's text became perhaps the most unread epitaph in herbal history (Thurston, 1900). The primary feature of H2.0 became the elimination of the author-expert as subject and object of herbal knowledge. The herbal was replaced by the monograph; Eminence Based Medicine was replaced by Evidence Based Medicine.

If the monograph first emerged in response to political assaults, it also remained, through successive iterations, the primary go-to means of deflecting or neutralising legal-regulatory initiatives intended to minimise the credibility of and availability of herbal medicines. Internally, botanical monographs vary in emphasis from the analytical and quality-oriented through phytopharmacological to the more therapeutic, but in essence the monographic description of a herb is based on *measurables*, i.e. objective scientific data. Compared to the epistemic model of H1.0, the defining features of medicinal herbs in H2.0 no longer reside in their capacities, nature or their power to do, but in *what* they do. Virtues were replaced by actions. (The occasionally arcane terminology of herbal 'actions' may have its provenance in a less reductionist past, but this is more etymological than substantive.) The primary scaffolding within which the monograph frames herb actions is in the final analysis based upon reductionist biomedical considerations, while even those disciplines with experiential origins such as pharmacognosy gradually became veneers on mainstream analytical chemistry and pharmacology. Meanwhile, features such as safety, toxicology and standardisation absent from H1.0 (except rarely in the discussion of potentially poisonous herbs) became obligatory standard elements of every monographic account of a herbal medicine.

Both sides of the pond

Historically, there was something of a divergence between developments on different sides of the Atlantic, here covered briefly only to illustrate cultural variations on our theme. In the US, the closure of the last Eclectic Medical School in 1934 marked the definitive end of a two decade-plus debacle following the publication of the Flexner Report, during which North American herbal medicine was effectively destroyed. Transplanted to England, and dogged by initial internecine rivalries, the herbal profession survived, albeit by a slender thread, even as it was eliminated in the US.

Despite finding some refuge in the nascent naturopathy movement, herbalism did not really resurface in America until reignited by the counter-cultural movement of the '60s. Then, in classic pioneer tradition, a handful of entrepreneurial individuals (aka hippies) began making and selling herbal extracts and giving classes on how to use them. Herbal education in the US still largely follows an apprenticeship model. There are dozens of schools and courses but no generally accepted core curriculum or educational standards, often with ad hoc scientific and minimal if any real medical training (excluding the handful of official naturopathic schools whose mixed menu curricula feature botanicals – amongst other things). This created something of a vacuum in terms of any substantive underlying philosophical and medical underpinnings of herbalism per se which results in some culturally unique curiosities. There is, for example, a tendency in North American herbalism for individuals to feel they have to 'invent' herbal 'systems' of their own. Notable examples include the late William Le Sassier's Triune System, and Southwestern herbalist Michael Moore's Clinical Energetics, and arguably could also include Michael Tierra's Planetary Herbalism, or more recently Donnie Yance's Eclectic Triphasic Medical System (ETMS). The same vacuum underscored the translation and publication of the Complete Commission E monographs by the American Botanical Council in 1998, which represented a high water mark of what could be called 'monograph madness' (Blumenthal *et al.* 1998). That importing these irrelevant regulatory documents from Germany could possibly be justified by suggesting they constituted a definitive model for the future foundation of US scientific herbal medicine, speaks volumes about the persistent subterranean aftershocks that followed the seismic destruction of H1.0 in the US.

In England, on the other hand, political pressures, always more muted (or perhaps just deceptively genteel), nonetheless impacted developments in the monograph 'ecosystem.' The rather short *British Herbal Pharmacopoeia* (BHP) therapeutic monographs that the Scientific Committee of the British Herbal Medicine Association started publishing in 1971 were largely a response to Parliament's Medicines Act of 1968, and the herbs included were described with the predictable focus on safety, quality and efficacy. However, the short therapeutic sections of the early BHP monographs were insightful commentaries based on a shared educational and clinical experience of the herb amongst the UK professional practitioners rather than lists of scientific studies. The earlier BHP is a quite refreshing read today compared to the encyclopaedic compilations of citations that pass for more recent monograph collections (BHMA 1983).

Internationally, regulatory imperatives increasingly supervened and came to dominate the herbal landscape toward the end of the 20th century especially in the EU. The response, once again as political reflex, was the weighty European Scientific Cooperative on Phytotherapy

(ESCOP) monograph series, a formidable compilation intended to create a pan-European scientific rationale for herbal medicines that remains a showpiece and archetype of the strengths and limits of monographic herbal explication and of the gulf between a scientific and more tradition-oriented phytotherapy (ESCOP 2003). In retrospect, European phytotherapy straddled the divide as best it could, with emeriti such as Rudolf Fritz Weiss attempting the increasingly difficult task of riding two horses simultaneously. Weiss should be singled out as an authoritative advocate for a theoretically coherent and unified (not integrative) concept of phytotherapy. Born in the 19th century, by 1985 already retired, he added a warning chapter to the sixth edition of his seminal *Lehrbuch der Phytotherapie* in which he painted a clairvoyant but detailed picture of the dangers of importing reductionist biomedical thinking into the phytotherapy that he had represented with nuance, deftness and refinement for so long. Weiss' essay, together with much of Thurston's 1900 *Philosophy of Physiomedicalism*, are arguably the most prescient and articulate theoretical contributions to the herbal literature (Weiss 1988, Thurston 1900).

Straw Man dates Aunt Sally[3]

Returning to our theme of the epistemic basis of the different paradigms, it was inevitable that the imperatives of the scientific monograph to reduce knowledge of the complexity of herbal therapeutics to pharmacologic actions and prescriber indications, while ignoring even the existence of underlying theoretical and philosophical assumptions involved, would sooner or later bite back. In various publications and other forms of herbal discourse, the initial uneasy tension between clinical expertise and scientific approaches increasingly became framed as an adversarial conflict between 'traditional knowledge' and reductionist biomedical science.

The actual definition of traditional knowledge (TK) approaches is likely to set the fur flying in debates among herbalists; in the interests of brevity, here I will list some of its generic features. TK tends to advocate and adhere to a 'whole plant' approach which is associated with several related core beliefs and principles of practice. Hence, TK pharmacy involves the use of whole herb, full spectrum extracts from fresh or dried herb material, usually as aqueous or hydroethanolic extracts. This is related to the belief that phytopharmacology is characterised by synergy between the multiple constituents of a plant, which in turn implies that isolated and concentrated 'active principles' are not 'true medicines'[4] but in reality ersatz pharmaceutical drugs. Whole plant ideology is often accompanied by a more 'earth-centered' or naturalistic worldview in which separation from nature and from folk knowledge of natural remedies is seen as the inevitable by-product of the defects in advanced technological culture. The 'whole plant' view tends be associated with espousal of 'wholism' in general (for example as in the 'whole person') as a credential. Further, it often places unnecessarily high (or politically correct) value on indigenous or ethnobotanical information, 'folk' traditions, and indeed shamanistic and spiritual approaches in which the plants are described as 'teachers'; the 'vitalist' epithet is often a short-hand descriptor identifying one or more of these proclivities.

Typically, the more strongly these positions are held, the more sharply are they opposed. *In extremis*, the hostile or negative views of biomedical science in this context tend toward a colouring book parody of science, wedded to ideological claims about science, ranging from it being an irrelevant and bankrupt materialist-reductionist delusion, through to conspiracy theories of science as a malefic tool of Big Pharma and corporate capitalism whose agenda is social control, including suppression of grass roots access to herbs – the science straw man. At the same time, traditional knowledge morphs into subcultural movements of a self-proclaimed 'folk' herbal renaissance that fights the good fight against the evils of professionalism, scientism and other 'very-bad-things' as Winnie the Pooh might say.

Metaphorically, we now have to get down with, not only the Straw Man, but with the Straw Man dating Aunt Sally. I would venture their best bet for a long term relationship and future happiness is therapeutic transformation of their caricature identities to transcend their otherwise historically limited estimated life span – or in what might here be dubbed a 'psychokuhnian check-in' in light of the increasingly obvious anomalous and incommensurable data that threaten to intrude on their frivolities. Detailing this process in-depth will have to wait until the second part of this article.

Here, I have proposed a conceptual foundation for articulating the historical trajectory of Western herbal medicine based upon the premise that its current paradigm is in a 'Kuhnian' crisis. The core of clinical herbal *medicine* is defined by its view of herbal *medicines*. The metaphysics of materia medica are the foundation of our medicine, as

Thurston and Weiss both clearly saw. Herbal medicine and modern biomedicine may have a shared phylogeny, but the key to understanding this was always the plants themselves. Today, preclinical and clinical science has progressed to a point well beyond its own '2.0,' but herbal medicine appears, like Gatsby, to be fighting for a future that tragically recedes into the past. Having set out some preliminary conceptual foundations here, a variety of lenses and tools will be employed in the next instalment, from literary criticism and integral philosophy to complexity theory, bioinformatics and network pharmacology. In Part 2, I will use this potpourri of approaches to argue in detail how a viable future Herbalism 3.0 requires restoring the primacy of materia medica by retooling the H1.0 concept of *natures* or *virtues* of herbs with the insights of 21st century life sciences.

References

BHMA, 1983. *British herbal pharmacopoeia*, Bournemouth: British Herbal Medicine Association.

Blumenthal, M., *et al.*, eds., 1998. *The complete German commission E monographs*. Austin: American Botanical Council: Integrative Medicine Communications.

European Scientific Cooperative On Phytotherapy, 2003. *ESCOP monographs*. Exeter: Thieme & European Scientific Cooperative on Phytotherapy.

Foster Wallace, D., 2009. *This is water: some thoughts, delivered on a significant occasion, about living a compassionate life*. New York: Little, Brown and Company.

Francia, S. and Stobart, A., eds., 2014. *Critical approaches to the history of Western herbal medicine*. London: Bloomsbury.

Tobyn G., Denham A. and Whitelegg M., 2011. *The Western herbal tradition: 2000 years of medicinal plant knowledge*. Edinburgh: Churchill Livingstone.

Griggs, B., 1981. *Green pharmacy the history and evolution of Western herbal medicine*. Vermont: Healing Arts Press.

Kuhn, T., 1962. *The structure of scientific revolutions*. Chicago: University of Chicago Press.

Thurston, J., 1900. *The philosophy of physiomedicalism*. Richmond, IA: Nicholson Printing and Manufacturing.

Weiss, R., 1988. *Herbal medicine*. 6th ed. Beaconsfield Publishers.

Notes

[1] I was first inspired by the profound utility of this field by Marxist philosophers Mary Hesse and Bob Young at Cambridge in the 1960s, but more recently have found the works of the feminist philosopher of science Evylyn Fox-Keller, and the Stanford School authors Nancy Cartwright and John Dupre invaluable in formulating my thoughts on H3.0 here, and beyond.

[2] Paraphrased from the definition of a true conservative attributed to W. Buckley.

[3] For US readers, Aunt Sally is a metaphorical English term, like Straw Man, denoting a fair ground game figure deliberately set up by someone in order to knock it down.

[4] Thurston's terminology for herbal medicines (true medicines) as opposed to pharmaceutical drugs which he classed as poison.

Biographies & Appendices

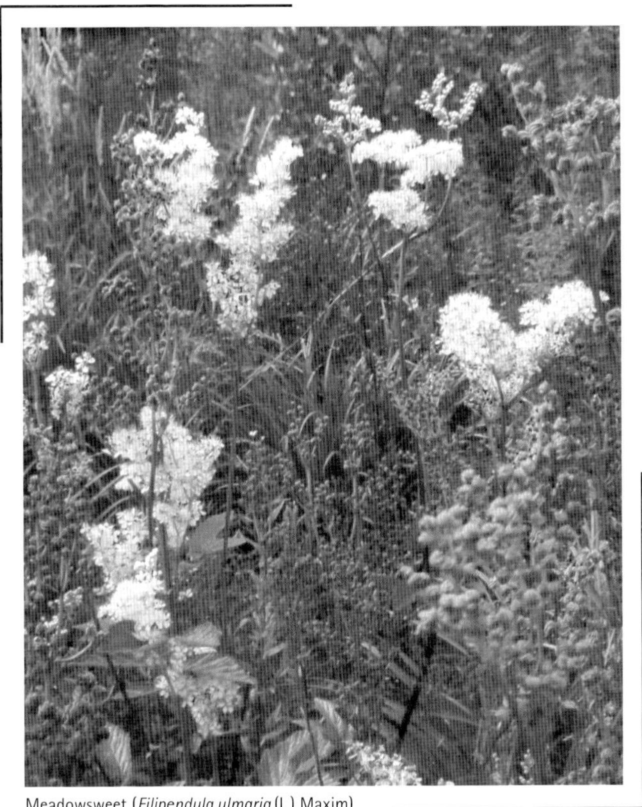

Meadowsweet (*Filipendula ulmaria* (L.) Maxim)

Biographies of Contributors

Dee Atkinson BSc(Hons) MNIMH

Dee studied at the School of Herbal Medicine in Tunbridge Wells in 1988 and started practising at Napiers of Edinburgh. A year later she took over the business and over the next 20 years, built the Napiers brand, at one time having 14 shops and clinics across the UK. The old recipes were re-established and new ones developed. Dee has held office on both councils of the College of Practitioners of Phytotherapy and the National Institute of Medical Herbalists (NIMH). She sat on the first Herbal Medicine Regulatory Working Group and is a member of the Herbal Forum. Dee has worked in radio and television promoting herbal medicine and has a busy practice in Edinburgh.

Julian Barker FLS Dip Phyt MCPP MNIMH

Julian Barker started his training in North and Central America, then returned to Britain as an apprentice herb-grower at Suffolk Herbs while studying concurrently on NIMH's tutorial course, before joining the first cohort at the School of Herbal Medicine. He became a member of NIMH in 1982 and opened a multidisciplinary clinic in Brighton, where he ran a training clinic until 2009. He has served on NIMH's Accreditation Board since 1998. Teaching Botany at the School of Herbal Medicine for over 20 years, Julian supervised BSc dissertations and taught Philosophy on the MSc course in herbal medicine at the University of East London. Since 1998 he has worked in Paris and studied in London with Dr Jean-Claude Lapraz on the application of medicinal plants along endobiogenic lines.

Kerry Bone BSc(Hons) Dip Phyto

Kerry Bone is co-founder and the innovation driver at MediHerb, a practising herbalist for 29 years, Director of Research and Development at MediHerb and Principal of the

Australian College of Phytotherapy. Kerry is also Adjunct Professor at New York Chiropractic College, providing input into their postgraduate applied nutrition programme. Kerry is a respected author of more than 30 scientific papers on herbal research, including original research and systematic reviews. He has also written or co-written six popular textbooks on herbal medicine, including his latest with Simon Mills, the long-awaited second edition of *Principles and Practice of Phytotherapy*, which was awarded the James A. Duke Excellence in Botanical Literature Award by the American Botanical Council in 2013.

Hananja Brice-Ytsma MSc DipEd DipTh MNIMH

Hananja has been practising herbal medicine for over 25 years. Qualified as a Naturopath in 1982 and then as a medical herbalist in 1990. In 1995, Hananja helped to pioneer Britain's first BSc degree in herbal medicine in partnership with Middlesex University. She lectures widely throughout the UK on gynaecology and paediatrics, and gives regular seminars on herbal medicine to GPs and medical consultants. Hananja has contributed to the BBC series and accompanying books *Grow Your Own Drugs* and is serving on NIMH council as Director of Education.

Chanchal Cabrera MSc FNIMH (RH)AHG

Chanchal has been a member of NIMH since 1987 and obtained her MSc in herbal medicine at the University of Wales in 2003. She was awarded a fellowship by NIMH in 2009 for more than 25 years service to the herbal profession. Chanchal's clinical specialty is helping people to manage cancer and chronic disease. She has held the faculty chair in Botanical Medicine at the Boucher Institute of Naturopathic Medicine, New Westminster since 2004. Chanchal serves on the Board of Advisors of the Dominion Herbal College in Burnaby, British Columbia and the editorial board of *Medical Herbalism* clinical newsletter. She publishes in professional journals and lectures internationally on medical herbalism, nutrition and health.

Paul Chenery PGDipHE MNIMH

Paul Chenery dropped out of studying biochemistry at Oxford as a teenager in 1969. After becoming a biodynamic organic farmer in the 1980s, he started growing medicinal herbs, qualifying in herbal medicine under Hein Zeylstra in 1999. A former Honorary General Secretary of NIMH, he is currently the UK representative to the European Herb Growers Association and a member of the UK Herbal Forum. He was appointed a Qualified Person by the MHRA in 2008 and is director of Rutland Biodynamics where he lives, farms and makes medicines under cGMP regulations.

Andrew Chevallier MCPP

Andrew trained at the School of Herbal Medicine in the 1980s, joining NIMH after qualifying from its tutorial course in 1986. For five years he worked (p/t) in an NHS-funded clinic in east London, providing herbal treatment to people over 55. He was Director of Education, Vice-President and then President of NIMH in the 1990s, becoming a fellow in 1997. Andrew helped to establish the first university-based degree in herbal medicine at Middlesex University in 1994, and as a senior lecturer taught materia medica and herbal therapeutics. He has written several books including *Encyclopaedia of Herbal Medicine, Herbal Medicine for the Menopause* and *Herbal Remedies.*

Peter Conway DipPhyt Cert Ed PGDip FCPP FNIMH

Peter is a Fellow of both the National Institute of Medical Herbalists and the College of Practitioners of Phytotherapy. He was President of the College of Practitioners of Phytotherapy from 2002 to 2012. His textbook *The Consultation in Phytotherapy* was published by Elsevier in 2011. Peter practises from his clinic in Tunbridge Wells where he has a special interest in working with complex and chronic conditions. He is currently a Visiting Professor at Pacific Rim College in Victoria, B.C., Canada.

Alison Denham MA FNIMH FHEA

Alison qualified as a herbalist in 1984, and is a former president of NIMH. Alison has published papers on the prescribing and the safety of medicinal plants, and is a member of the Herbal Medicines Advisory Committee of the UK Medicines and Healthcare products Regulatory Agency. Alison was part of a team which ran a pilot randomised controlled study on the care of women during the menopause by herbal practitioners. Alison teaches on the e-learning MSc in herbal medicine at the University of Central Lancashire and this year completed her postgraduate research on John Skelton (1805–1880) a prominent Chartist and leading herbal practitioner.

Jan de Vries ND MRN DHomMed MBAcA DSc(Hon)

Jan was born in Kampen, Holland on 26th January 1937. Graduating in pharmacy in 1958, Jan changed direction early in his career following a chance meeting with Dr Alfred Vogel in 1960 and after studying homoeopathy with him in Switzerland, they continued to work together for 35 years. Jan has written over 40 books including *The Female Cancers: a Complementary Approach.* Jan has lectured at seminars, conferences and universities throughout the world and helped develop natural medicine in India, Canada, Australia, America and Scandinavia. In 2002 Jan was made an honorary professor of the Queen Margaret

University College in Edinburgh in recognition of his entrepreneurial activities in the field of naturopathic medicine.

Dr Michael Dixon OBE MA FRCGP

Michael Dixon graduated in psychology and philosophy from Oxford University before studying medicine at Guy's Hospital. He has been a GP in Cullompton, Devon since 1984. He is chair of NHS Alliance; Visiting Professor at the University of Westminster; Honorary Senior Fellow in Public Policy at the Health Services Management Centre, University of Birmingham; and Honorary Senior Lecturer in Integrated Health at the Peninsula Medical School. He is also a Senior Associate at the King's Fund where he is a member of the Steering Group of the Inquiry into quality of GP care. He was the medical director of The Prince's Foundation for Integrated Health. In 2010, he was elected chair of The College of Medicine.

Serene Foster DPhil (Oxon) BSc(Hons) BSc(Hons) MBSI MNIMH MCPP

Serene Foster is a senior Medical Immunologist and has been associated with Hydes Herbal Clinic since 1997. She has been Principal Herbal Practitioner, working full time, since 2003. Serene is a registered member of the British Society of Immunologists and specialises in Autoimmunity, Viral Immunology, Transplantation Immunology, respiratory medicine and allergy. She has worked at The John Radcliffe Hospital, University of Oxford, The Imperial Cancer Research Fund, London, Imperial College School of Medicine at St Mary's, London and Immunotoxicology in Leicester.

Jane Gray DipPhyt Cert Ed FNIMH

Jane began her study of herbal medicine at the College of Phytotherapy in 1996. At this time she became a student affiliate of NIMH and helped catalogue material given to the institute by Fred Fletcher Hyde and this was the beginning of Jane's longtime interest in the NIMH Library. Jane joined NIMH in 2000 as a practising member and in 2003, was invited on to the Accreditation Board and shortly after, appointed Accreditation Officer. For the next decade Jane had successive roles in NIMH as Director of Education, Vice President, President and Honorary General Secretary. Jane is chair of the Library Committee and continues to practise as a medical herbalist in Stockport, Manchester.

Barbara Griggs

Barbara has been researching and writing about herbs, health, nutrition and natural medicine for nearly 40 years. The many books she has published include *Green Pharmacy: a*

History of Western Herbal Medicine, widely regarded as the definitive work on the subject and more recently *Helpful Herbs for Health and Beauty*. Barbara was Health Editor of *Country Living* for nineteen years from its launch in 1986. In 2005 the NIMH elected her an Honorary Associate in recognition of a long and distinguished career in the service of herbal medicine. Barbara has often appeared on radio and television, and lectured on herbal medicine at international conferences in the UK, USA and Australia.

Frances Hambly MNIMH

Frances graduated from the School of Herbal Medicine, Tunbridge Wells in 1987 and practises in East Sussex where she runs a herbal clinic and dispensary with husband and medical herbalist, Paul Hambly. Frances has two children and is committed to natural ways of raising children and treating childhood illnesses. Frances is the author of *Herbal Medicine for Children* and co-author of *Herbalism*. She studied Aromatic Medicine with Dr Daniel Penoel in1992–1993 and completed the GAPS (gut and psychology syndrome) practitioner training in 2013. Frances is also an external examiner for the final clinical exams on the Herbal Medicine BSc degree at Middlesex University and mentors newly qualified NIMH members.

Christopher Hedley AHG

Christopher Hedley qualified with the National Institute of Medical Herbalists' School of Herbal Medicine in 1982. He served on NIMH council and on the Postgraduate Training Board amongst other duties. He was awarded a fellowship of the Institute in 1999. He is currently a member of the American Herbalist Guild and in private practice in London. Christopher has taught herbal medicine at all levels from beginners to MSc and is known for his informative but relaxed style.

Fred Fletcher Hyde BSc FNIMH

President Emeritus both of NIMH and also of the British Herbal Medicine Association, Fred had a degree in Chemistry and first class honours in Botany from London University. He was founder of the Education Fund and the School of Herbal Medicine. A former member of the committee on Review of Medicines and was responsible for herbal medicine having a place in the Statute Book (Medicines Act 1968). For 16 years he was chairman of the British Herbal Pharmacopoeia; entered NAMH in 1931 and directed the Research and Analytical Department for 50 years.

Robyn James BA(Oxon) MNIMH Cert Phyt

Robyn trained as a herbalist with the School of Phytotherapy in the mid-1990s. She established 'Alton and James' a herbal shop, clinic and public dispensary in Sheffield in October 2000 and continues to practise as a medical herbalist from the same premises. Robyn previously taught at the College of Phytotherapy and as a supervisor at the herbal training clinic of the University of Central Lancashire. She is now a senior lecturer on the Lincoln BSc(Hons) Herbal Medicine course. Robyn also has many years of experience volunteering at and running festival clinics that provide acute herbal medicine and first aid and is now a partner in a travelling festival sauna.

Marion Mackonochie BSc(Hons) MNIMH

After a first degree in pharmacology and physiology and a few years editing science journals, Marion retrained in herbal medicine at Middlesex University, where she achieved a first. She continues to edit science journals and is copy editor for the *Journal of Herbal Medicine*, as well as being a practising herbalist in Brighton, and is in the process of opening up a herbal shop and information centre with two other herbalists to promote access to herbal medicine. Marion has trained in endobiogenics with Jean-Claude Lapraz and is particularly interested in hormonal issues.

Michael McIntyre MA FNIMH MRCHM MCPP MBAcC DUniv

Michael McIntyre has practised herbal medicine and acupuncture for over 30 years in the Cotswolds. He has chaired the European Herbal and Traditional Medicines Practitioner Association since its launch in 1993. He has an honorary doctorate from Middlesex University and is currently a visiting Professor there. He is a fellow and life member of NIMH as well as a former president of the Institute. Michael regularly writes, lectures and broadcasts on herbal medicine as well as on regulation of this sector. In 2014 he gave evidence in person to the House of Commons Select Committee on Science and Technology inquiry into antimicrobial resistance.

Kevin Orbell-McSean MNIMH

Kevin graduated from the School of Herbal Medicine in 1989, after many years of informal learning from his grandfather and medical herbalist Albert Orbell FNIMH. Shortly after graduating he set up practice in Cork, Ireland. Kevin was one of the first qualified medical herbalists to practise in Ireland, and a founding member and inaugural president of the Irish Association of Medical Herbalists, now known as the Irish Institute of Medical Herbalists (IIMH). He served on the NIMH Professional Ethics Working Group from 2005-2009.

Today, Kevin lectures to undergraduate and postgraduates, hosts clinical hours training at his clinic and mentors newly qualified herbalists joining NIMH.

Keith Robertson MSc FNIMH

Keith is a visionary and pioneer of traditional energetic and contemplative approaches in professional herbal training in the UK. After serving on the NIMH council he established the Scottish School of Herbal Medicine in Glasgow with his wife Maureen in 1992. They were inspired by Goethe's work and for 18 years trained herbal students to BSc and MSc level. In recognition of Keith's vision of SSHM, as well as his work with NIMH and EHPTA Accreditation Boards, Keith was made a fellow in 2004 for his services to herbal education. Keith has been a practising medical herbalist since 1989 and runs a herbal correspondence course and apprenticeship programme from the herb farm on the Isle of Arran.

Caroline Sheldrick BA(Hons) BSc(Hons) Cert Ed MNIMH

As a very mature student, Caroline completed her herbal medicine training at Middlesex University in 2003 and has been a full-time herbalist in rural Gloucestershire since 2013. Most of her previous career has been in non-fiction publishing, as an editor of educational, academic and medical publications. Caroline is currently studying the physical and mental health effects of traumatic stress.

Desiree Shelley BSc(Hons) MNIMH

Desiree trained as a Registered General Nurse at Addenbrookes Hospital in Cambridge, and then as a Registered Health Visitor in Ipswich. She worked as a Health Visitor, then Team Leader and then a Community Services manager. In 1997 she started the distance learning degree course at the College of Phytotherapy, East Sussex and became a full NIMH member on graduating from the University of Wales. Desiree was co-opted on to the NIMH Council in 2007. She was elected president of NIMH in 2010 and served for three years. Desiree is currently researching the history of NIMH with a view to publishing a book in due course.

Laura Stannard BA(Hons) Dip Phyt FNIMH

Laura joined NIMH after graduating from the College of Phytotherapy in 1994. She was co-opted on to the NIMH Council in 1996 and was Director of Education from 1997 to 2001. Laura returned to the NIMH Council in 2006 and has been PR Director (briefly), Chair of the Postgraduate Training Board, Director of Professional Development and Vice

President, becoming President in 2013. Laura practised in clinics in Taunton and Chard in Somerset for fifteen years, including several years at Warwick House Medical Centre in Taunton, before re-locating to the southernmost tip of Cheshire in 2009. She practises close to Stoke on Trent.

Anne Stobart BSc PhD MNIMH

As a medical herbalist, organic gardener and teacher, Anne has fulfilled a lifelong passion for working with plants. After developing her clinical practice in Devon, she taught professional herbal medicine based at Middlesex University in London, where she was Director of Programmes for Complementary Health Sciences until 2010. Her interest in women's health and medical history led to a doctoral thesis on the use of medicinal receipts in early modern domestic medicine. Anne has published on domestic medicine and co-edited *Critical Approaches to the History of Western Herbal Medicine*. She is an Honorary Research Fellow at the University of Exeter and co-founder of the Herbal History Research Network and the Holt Wood Herbs Project in North Devon.

Graeme Tobyn BA PGDipHE FHEA FNIMH

Graeme joined NIMH after graduating from the School of Herbal Medicine with the Arthur Barker prize in 1990. During 24 years' practice he has worked as a herbalist in the NHS and as a clinical tutor in a number of herbal training clinics. He was appointed senior lecturer at UCLan in 2000, and became course leader of herbal medicine. Graeme has lectured and acted as clinical examiner at several herbal training and postgraduate programmes in the UK. He is now course leader for the online MSc herbal medicine programme at UCLan and was awarded a NIMH fellowship in 2007. He is co-author of *The Western Herbal Tradition* and is completing a PhD at Lancaster University in the history of medicine.

Jonathan Treasure MA MNIMH RH(AHG)

Jonathan graduated in medical sciences at Cambridge University, and later trained at the UK School of Phytotherapy. An Oregon resident for the last twenty years, his clinical practice combines botanicals with cutting-edge oncology in personalised cancer treatment strategies. He is a member of the American Herbalist Guild and the Society of Integrative Oncology. He is author of the herb section of the collaborative *Herb, Drug, Nutrient Interactions: Clinical Implications and Therapeutic Strategies* and is currently writing a book *Cannabis and Cancer.* 'Herbalism 3.0' is a work-in-progress created to mark the dual anniversaries in 2014 of both the AHG (25th) and the NIMH (150th).

Ruth Trickey ND Medical Herbalist

Ruth Trickey has worked as a medical herbalist in Melbourne, Australia for the past 34 years. She specialises in the treatment of gynaecological complaints and is currently working collaboratively with fertility specialists at Melbourne IVF to optimise the treatment of women with premature ovarian failure. She is the author of *Women, Hormones and the Menstrual Cycle*.

Frances Watkins BSc(Hons) PhD MCPP MNIMH

Frances graduated from Middlesex University in 2009 with a first class honours in herbal medicine after more than 20 years in marketing and public relations. She completed her doctorate in 2013 at the University of East London investigating native British plants used in 10th century Anglo-Saxon wound healing formulations. During this time Frances published papers in *Drug Discovery Today* and the *Journal of Ethnopharmacology*. She is a practising medical herbalist in Watford, Herts and is interested in menopause and executive stress.

Julie Whitehouse BSc(Hons) PhD MCPP

Julie has been a practising medical herbalist and a teacher of herbal medicine for over 20 years. She is a principal lecturer at the University of Westminster and programme leader of the BSc honours degree in herbal medicine. Her research interests, shared with the members of the herbal research team at University of Westminster include the use of skullcap for treatment of anxiety and mood enhancement, herbal bitters and caffeine on digestive and cardiovascular physiology and the professional practice and patient experience of Western herbal medicine.

Hein Zeylstra MCPP

Principal of the School of Phytotherapy (herbal medicine) and Editor-in-Chief of the *British Journal of Phytotherapy*. He practised as a medical herbalist for about 20 years, and was involved for 40 years in the commercial production of botanical drugs and the manufacture of herbal preparations. He was one of the two members for the United Kingdom on the Scientific Committee of ESCOP (European Scientific Cooperative for Phytotherapy).

Appendix 1: Abbreviations

AHG	American Herbalists Guild
(RH) AHG	Registered Herbalist with American Herbalist Guild
BSc(Hons)	Bachelor of Science with honours
CAM	Complementary and Alternative Medicine
Cert Ed	Certificate of Education
CNC	Clinic for Natural Healing
CPP	College of Practitioners of Phytotherapy
DIHom	Diploma in Homeopathy
Dip Ed	Diploma in Education
Dip Phyt	Diploma in Phytotherapy
Dip Th	Diploma in Applied Theology
EHTPA	European Herbal and Traditional Practitioners Association
FHEA	Fellow of Higher Education Academy
FLS	Fellow of the Linnean Society
FNIMH	Fellow of NIMH
HE	Higher Education
HNH	Hospital for Natural Healing
IIMH	Irish Institute of Medical Herbalists
MA	Master of Arts
MSc	Master of Science
MBAcC	Member of the British Acupuncture Council
MCPP	Member of CPP
MNIMH	Member of NIMH
MRCHM	Member of the Register of Chinese Herbal Medicine
MRN	Member of the Register of Naturopaths
NAMH	National Association of Medical Herbalists
ND	Naturopathic Doctor

NIMH	National Institute of Medical Herbalists
PGDip	Post Graduate Diploma
PhD	Doctor of Philosophy
SSHM	Scottish School of Herbal Medicine

Appendix 2: The National Institute of Medical Herbalists (NIMH)

The National Institute of Medical Herbalists was established in 1864 and is the oldest body of practising herbalists in existence today. NIMH is made up of:

Members
Fellows
Life Members
Honorary Associates
Student Affiliates

NIMH members can be recognised by the letters MNIMH or FNIMH after their name.

A copy of the NIMH Register of Qualified Members may be obtained by sending an A5 self-addressed envelope to:

Honorary General Secretary
The National Institute of Medical Herbalists
Clover House
James Court
South Street
Exeter
Devon EX1 1EE

For more information about NIMH please telephone (01392) 426022, email info@nimh.org.uk or visit the website at http://www.nimh.org.uk

The NIMH publishes the *Journal of Herbal Medicine* in collaboration with the international publishing house, Elsevier. It focuses on the profession and practice of herbal medicine and contains profession related material in the form of case studies, original research articles, reviews, monographs, clinical trials and relevant in vitro studies.
Visit: http://ees.elsevier.com/hermed/

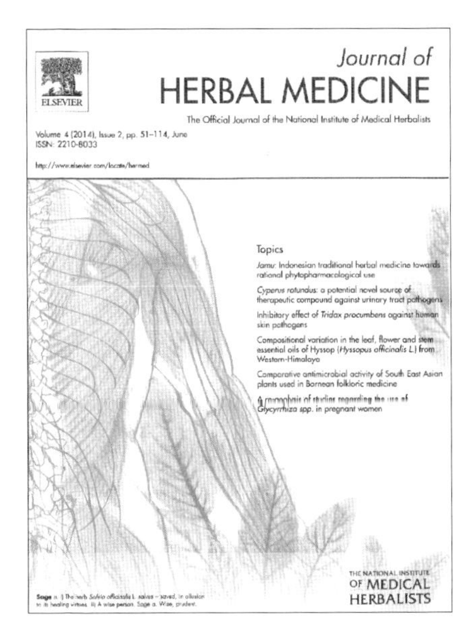

Appendix 3: Presidents of the National Institute of Medical Herbalists (1864-2014)

Name	Year
Dr John Skelton (Jnr)	(1864–1866)
Dr J P Payne	(1866–1867)
Mr William Blunt	(1870s–1880s)
Mr Goodwin	(1886–1887)
Mr Alfred R. Fox	(1890–1896)
Mr Samuel Halliday	(1896–1901)
Mr James Parkinson	(1901–1907)
Mr James. W. Scurrah	(1907–1912)
Mr John Marlow	(1912–1917)
Mr Korah Culpan	(1917–1921)
Mr W. Burns Lingard	(1921–1924)
Mr Joseph Watmore	(1924–1930)
Mr William Dawes	(1930–1934)
Mr Arthur Barker	(1934–1937)
Mr Tom Hunter	(1937–1939)
Mr Arthur Barker	(1939–1952)
Mr W. T. Hewitt	(1952–1954)
Mr Ernest Cockayne	(1954–1957)
Mr Horace Mansfield	(1957–1958)
Mr W. Burns Lingard	(1958–1960)
Mr Frank Crosswaite	(1960–1961)
Mr C. Wilfred Morley	(1961–1963)
Mr Albert Orbell	(1963–1965)
Mr Arthur Jenner	(1965–1968)
Mr Fred Fletcher Hyde	(1968–1975)*
Mrs Nalda Gosling	(1975–1978)
Mr John D. Hyde	(1978–1980)
Mr Eric Robson	(1980–1982)
Mr Simon Mills	(1982–1988)
Ms Kristin Jeffs	(1988–1990)
Mr Simon Mills	(1990–1991)
Mr Mark Evans	(1991–1992)
Mr Michael McIntyre	(1992–1994)
Mr Andrew Chevallier	(1994–1996)
Ms Christine Steward	(1996–1998)
Mrs Midge Whitelegg	(1998–2000)
Ms Alison Denham	(2000–2002)
Ms Trudy Norris	(2002–2004)
Mr Ned Reiter	(2004–2006)
Mr Steve Kippax	(2006–2008)
Mrs Jane Gray	(2008–2010)
Mrs Desiree Shelley	(2010–2013)
Mrs Laura Stannard	(2013–)

* Awarded the honorary title of President Emeritus by NIMH in 1968

Appendix 4: Credits

In addition to the plant photographs taken by Kay Piercy to illustrate the sections within the book, NIMH would like to thank the following for their kind permission to reproduce their photographs and diagrams:

Dee Atkinson – John Napier preparing tinctures (p.13), Mrs Meekins (p.14)

Serene Foster – Hydes Herbal Clinic in St. Peter's Road Leicester (p.40), Hydes dispensary (p.42), Fred Fletcher Hyde and John Hyde (p.45)

Kevin Orbell McSean – Hospital for Natural Healing (p.36), HNH Student Group in 1950s (p.37), Albert Orbell explaining different preparations (p.38),

Ruth Trickey – Treatment algorithm for ROS/POF (p.170)

Jonathan Treasure – Fig 1. Graphic representation of Khunian science (p.236), Fig 2. Graphic timeline of Khunian paradigms in Western herbal history (p.237)

The Plant List database, a collaboration between the Royal Botanic Gardens, Kew and Missouri Botanical Garden has been used to confirm the plant authorities used in this book. http://www.theplantlist.org

Index

Please note, page numbers in *italics* refer to illustrations, and those in **bold** type, to a table.

Q

R

S

T